# Watercolor Bedroom

## Creating a Soulful Midlife

By

Daphne Stevens, Ph.D.

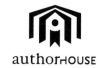

authorHOUSE

*1663 LIBERTY DRIVE, SUITE 200*
*BLOOMINGTON, INDIANA 47403*
*(800) 839-8640*
*www.authorhouse.com*

© 2004 Daphne Stevens, Ph.D.
All Rights Reserved.

No part of this book may be reproduced, stored in a retrieval system, or transmitted by any means without the written permission of the author.

First published by AuthorHouse 09/02/04

ISBN: 1-4184-0887-5 (e)
ISBN: 1-4184-0886-7 (sc)


Library of Congress Control Number: 2004091894

Printed in the United States of America
Bloomington, Indiana

This book is printed on acid-free paper.

# Acknowledgements

I want to express my gratitude to the following people:

To my parents, David and Juanita Stevens, who launched me into a love of words.

To my daughter, Carson Anne Leegate, whose courage, compassion, and creativity are an ongoing source of wonder to me.

To Barbara Nance, in whose truth-telling love I have learned to celebrate each phase of my life.

To Lisa Groen Baner, for generous support in the writing process, and for email conversations that continue to inspire me.

To Jean Marriott, who responded to my words with images and colors, a loving brushstroke for every keystroke, to create beautiful cover art.

To Dan and Linda Edwards, for cherished companionship, spiritual wisdom, and endless evenings of shared hospitality.

To Donna Groover and Beth West, healers and kindred spirits who have deepened my understanding of what family means.

To Kristina Simms and to Linda Edwards for generous and painstaking editing efforts.

To Heather Pritchard, whose organizational skills and eye for beauty have been invaluable in keeping me focused.

To my community at St. Francis Episcopal Church for a diverse and inclusive safe haven of spiritual growth and exploration.

To Fay Key, Steve Bullington, and Gail Pitt of Green Bough House of Prayer, for a welcoming place for prayer and meditation.

To Drs. Cindy Carter and Dianne Skafte and the community of Pacifica Graduate Institute, for nurturing places where Soul can be tended.

To my circle of wise women friends in Macon, Georgia, and to the clients who have entrusted me with their stories and dreams through the years.

And, finally, thanks to Aaron Bowers, with whose enthusiastic support rooms are built and visions are conceived and birthed.

For Aaron,

my two-hanky gentleman

with great admiration and love

# Table of Contents

Acknowledgements .................................................................... iii
Prologue .................................................................................... ix
Chapter 1: Grandmother God ................................................... 1
Chapter 2: Watercolor Bedroom ............................................... 5
Chapter 3: Feeding the Muse .................................................... 9
Chapter 4: Creating a Vision ................................................... 12
Chapter 5: Snakes and Angels ................................................. 17
Chapter 6: Demeter's Daughter ............................................... 22
Chapter 7: Dream-Tending ...................................................... 28
Chapter 8: Changing Careers .................................................. 32
Chapter 9: Ash Wednesday ..................................................... 37
Chapter 10: A Pink Blanket of Love ....................................... 40
Chapter 11: Showing Up .......................................................... 46
Chapter 12: Staying Awake ..................................................... 51
Chapter 13: Telling the Truth .................................................. 56
Chapter 14: Letting Go ............................................................ 61
Chapter 15: Easter Morning ..................................................... 65
Chapter 16: Unfinished Children ............................................. 70
Chapter 17: Radical Self-Care ................................................. 74
Chapter 18: Holy Commerce ................................................... 78
Chapter 19: Mother's Day ....................................................... 82
Chapter 20: Dancing Lessons .................................................. 87
Chapter 21: Sweet Melancholy ............................................... 92
Chapter 22: Pleading Guilty .................................................... 96
Chapter 23: Words Fail ......................................................... 101
Chapter 24: Playing Hooky ................................................... 105
Chapter 25: Hot Flash ............................................................ 109
Chapter 26: Money Talks ...................................................... 113

Chapter 27: Midlife Goddess ........................................................... 117
Chapter 28: Brain Building ............................................................. 120
Chapter 29: Clearing Clutter ........................................................... 124
Chapter 30: Empty Nest .................................................................. 127
Chapter 31: Unfulfilled Hopes ........................................................ 131
Chapter 32: Time Away ................................................................... 135
Chapter 33: The Language of Complaint ...................................... 138
Chapter 34: Parking Lot Sacraments ............................................. 144
Chapter 35: Sensible Shoes ............................................................ 148
Chapter 36: Autumn's Kiss ............................................................. 152
Chapter 37: Political Wife .............................................................. 156
Chapter 38: Strong Bones ............................................................... 160
Chapter 39: The Essential No ......................................................... 164
Chapter 40: Sponges and Mirrors ................................................... 169
Chapter 41: The Third Woman ....................................................... 174
Chapter 42: Silent Retreat ............................................................... 179
Chapter 43: The Difference between Men and Women ................ 183
Chapter 44: Giving Thanks ............................................................. 188
Chapter 45: Kitchen Work .............................................................. 191
Chapter 46: Anger Management .................................................... 195
Chapter 47: The Long Road Toward Goodbye .............................. 201
Chapter 48: Accidental Joy ............................................................. 206
Chapter 49: Ficus Tree .................................................................... 210
Chapter 50: Christmas Week .......................................................... 214
Chapter 51: Birth Announcement ................................................... 217
Chapter 52: Wise Blood .................................................................. 221
Resources ........................................................................................ 224

# Prologue

Sometimes when I'm out doing everyday errands, I meet the eyes of a midlife woman. She's beleaguered by problems, or she's content. She's old before her time, or she's youthful and energetic. When we see one another, there's a spark of recognition.

"Don't I know you?" one of us may ask. Living in a small town means that we may very well have met each another, but the connection seems to go deeper than that.

"Midlife" has been used in the chronological sense—the midpoint in the life span, perhaps in our forties or fifties —but midlife is also the *center* of life. We stand at the crossroads between past and future, an intersection from which we can look forward and back with equal clarity of vision. We also stand at a tipping-point, a place from which we either come home to ourselves more fully or we succumb to despair and invisibility.

Our notions of midlife have been blurred by the fact that history has never known a generation of women who are healthier, more conscious, more educated, and more open to possibility than we are. We are the most vivacious creatures on the planet right now—but we can't claim that vitality unless we see midlife as the crucial and exciting developmental time that it is.

We grow into our authority to be ourselves through the realization of ten developmental tasks:

1. To create a vision for the second half of our lives—relationships, personal growth, spiritual fulfillment, physical environment—and take concrete action toward living into that vision.

2. To set appropriate boundaries with grown children and aging parents, while remaining available to them in loving ways.

3. To appreciate the physical and emotional changes of the menopausal years in order to fully optimize our health and well-being.

4. To explore our dreams and our inner lives more deeply so we can claim our spiritual birthright.

5. To step into our roles as elders in our families and communities with joy, dignity, and passion.

6. To rehearse for retirement by remembering the things we love to do and by exploring new uses of leisure time.

7. To identify the things that drain our energy and sort out the essential from the non-essential.

8. To develop a communication style that is clean, straightforward, and gracious in order to keep friendships and love relationships simple and nurturing.

9. To forge a relationship to issues of finitude and mortality that come into focus at this time of life.

10. To learn to lighten up, to play, and to delight in our sensual selves.

These ten tasks are the guide-lines for this book. As I wrote, I found myself moving from theories and directives into the realm of stories and intuitive links. I began to notice the experiences of everyday life as invitations to see the tasks of midlife, not as things to be accomplished but as truths that unfold like the petals of a flower, revealing ever-deepening color and fragrance to anyone who will slow down long enough to notice.

*Watercolor Bedroom* is devoted to the idea that, in being faithful to the work of caring for ourselves, we bless the larger community in some ineffable yet palpable way that can't otherwise happen. Both self-care and service to others are part of the evolution that happens in the day-to-day, seemingly insignificant choices we make as individual women. As we honor our bodies and feed our souls and spark our imaginations and listen to our dreams, we are truly tending the soul of the world.

This book is a collection of "snapshot" essays, each of which can be read in five minutes or less. Each chapter can be read as an independent piece, or the whole book can be read in progression, perhaps weekly, with accompanying journal work. Through the Questions for Reflection at the end of each chapter, you are encouraged to deepen into you own inner dialogue. What are the insights that connect this particular chapter with the themes of your life? How can you more consciously celebrate your own wisdom? And how can you more fully share what you know with the world?

*Watercolor Bedroom* is dedicated to the notion that each woman needs and deserves a womb-like matrix—a "watercolor bedroom" of her own design, where she can incubate the secrets of her soul and bring them into outward and visible forms to be celebrated and shared. Through this writing, I invite you to create that matrix and explore the mysteries that will be revealed to you there.

Daphne Stevens

# Chapter 1: Grandmother God

When I was a child, I studied the faces of women I knew. I saw them as young or old. "Young" meant unmarried and free, but it didn't seem particularly fun-loving or adventurous. "Old" meant alone and close to death, wearing the ravages of disease and deterioration with varying degrees of dignity. It never seemed wise or peaceful.

"Middle-aged" was a nondescript, pejorative term. "The bloom is off the magnolia," I heard someone say when I was a girl. No one had to explain the meaning. To cling to the "bloom" was a woman's only (albeit fragile and temporary) hope. To relinquish the dewy-eyed freshness of youth was to step straight into the jaws of decline and despair.

Women tried to be flippant as they voiced their fears. "At my age…" the line began. What followed was always something self-disparaging. "You're not getting older, you're getting better" sang a commercial for hair dye, preying on collective fears: Were we really doomed to that ultimate and horrible fate, just getting old? Was there a way to fight it? How could we exist without a fresh ingénue face to make us appealing to the world?

I now understand what I was seeking as a child when I searched the faces of those women. I was looking for a face that was filled with something other than anxiety about itself. I was looking for a face that reflected something about fully belonging—about knowing its own wisdom, about exuding a sense of graciousness in a world that is fraught with adolescent dramas and power struggles. I was looking for a face that would share its secrets with other women. I was looking for the face of midlife.

I didn't plan on wearing that face. I secretly held the hope that my spiritual quest would camouflage my fears and insulate me from a world that was bewildering in its competitiveness and cruelty. But three things happened as I slogged through school and pursued a career as a psychotherapist: One, I was transformed by the words of the poets who had transcended the wounds of time and ordinariness that seemed to doom my own young life. Two, as I listened to the stories I heard during the psychotherapy hour, I realized that the wisdom of the poet and the prophet often comes disguised in the words of ordinary people. And three, as I grew older, I continued searching the faces of women—now the faces of my peers. As they aged, some got resigned and bitter, or overly attached to that perpetual girlishness that borders on desperation. But in many of my women friends of all different ages, I saw glimpses of what I came to think of as Grandmother God.

Grandmother God for me embodied a timeless divine femininity, able to embrace both joy and sorrow, to be on the planet for her own sake alone, to be fierce without apology, and to love others fully because she had taken the perilous and courageous path of self-love. Grandmother God was generous for the sheer pleasure of it. I experienced her as I shared birthdays and wedding celebrations and births and deaths with my friends. I recognized her in the moment when one companion said, "You should buy that sweater. It's delicious against the color of your skin," and I heard her voice when another friend said, "Stop. Listen to yourself. This dream is telling you something." I felt her presence, too, in long solitary walks in the woods and on the beach—a presence at once encouraging and challenging, who could whisper words like, "You don't have to get it right all the time, honey," and at the same time not let me settle for anything less than the most authentic life I could live.

Grandmother God, too, could laugh at herself. She could see her own inner inconsistencies and view the foibles of others without judgment or criticism. In short, Grandmother God could have a good time. She could dance the dance of one who lives in a less-than-perfect body and sing her songs in a less-than-perfect-voice. And because she was less than perfect, she could invite others to sing and dance along with her—with the abandonment and sparkle that can only be shared by ordinary people in ordinary moments.

The truth, of course, is that we either despair or we become the images we long for. While I know I don't fully inhabit the world of Grandmother God, I know I am onto something because she inhabits my world. While I don't fully know how to get from "young" to "old" in a way that invites life and wisdom and peace, I know that midlife is a time, not only of transition, but of initiation into something rich and real.

I know, too, that experiences of insight and poetry usually come to us disguised as mundane moments. In our youth, we are taught to look for the Big Idea—the "Aha" moment that will make our lives fall into place. In midlife, we learn something about simply waking up, about being present to the Divine who sings within our dreams and speaks to us through the words of ordinary people.

"All sickness is homesickness," says the healer and author Dianne M. Connelly. And all healing is homecoming. Midlife is for healing— for coming home to the place in ourselves where Grandmother God waits with open arms.

Questions for Reflection:

1. What are the words or images that come to you as you reflect on the words, "Old," "Young," "Middle-Aged?"

2. Who are the role models—either people in your personal life, or those whose work and writing you've admired—that provide you with an image of mature womanhood?

Jot these down in your journal. Notice them as they show up in your dreams or in your day-to-day life. They are the "Grandmother Gods—" your inner guides for creating a soulful midlife.

# Chapter 2: Watercolor Bedroom

It all started when we drove into the driveway one day. In an offhand remark, I said to my husband, "This house has no curb appeal. It's inviting when we get inside. The living room is comfortable, the dining room is elegant. The kitchen is a great gathering place —but let's face it, Babe, from the outside we look pretty bleak."

My husband was inclined to agree with me. (He's usually inclined to agree with me.) So he hired a landscape architect who took a bunch of pictures and made a bunch of sketches—but the gist of his advice was, "Hey, your roof looks like hell."

Now, why did I never notice that? So we called a roofer who, upon inspection, discovered our house was weighed down by seven layers of shingles. No wonder the roof looked shabby. We decided to have him tear it all down and re-roof the house in a proper way.

Then the rains came. In the middle of a six-year drought, we were hit with the worst thunderstorm in history. Our denuded roof dripped the monsoons—sieve-like— straight through the ceilings into our rooms. I found my husband sitting in his office under an umbrella one day, the saddest man I've ever seen. So then there were ceilings to fix.

When we moved the furniture out to accommodate the ceiling-repair, we realized how bad the flooring looked. "While we're at it, we might as well refinish these floors." I thought longingly back to the days when I thought I was going to hire a landscape architect to help me with a master plan for the flower beds out front. I sighed. "Yes, let's fix the floors."

Well, floors are no good if the walls are in bad shape. And we had planned to install a French door to replace the out-dated patio door in the guest room anyway. What better time to install the new door than when the furniture is out and the floors are being re-done? And what better time to wallpaper the room than when the new French door has been installed? "What do you really want in this room?" my husband asked pleasantly.

At that point, my last nerve was gone. "I want a retreat! I want a room where I can go to escape from the roofing guys and the flooring guys and the ceiling guys and the French door guys! I want a room to get away from YOU when I need to!" It was the first real decision I had made in weeks, and it felt pretty good to get it out of my system.

So I trooped to the wallpaper store. "I want a watercolor bedroom," I announced. "I want a room that's soft and welcoming. A room with an air of feminine charm without any hint of dripping old-lady wisteria or perky little-girl rosebuds . I want a pastel room that doesn't look like an Easter basket or somebody's baby nursery. A room that can smell like rose or lavender or sage, depending on my mood. I want comfort and pleasure where I can read poetry and rest and primp and enjoy my hot flashes in peace."

The young salesperson looked perplexed. Anyone under the age of forty-five who hasn't read *A Room of One's Own* at least three times would be confused—but, to her credit, she got my drift.

*Watercolor Bedroom*

Every midlife woman needs a watercolor bedroom. Visions and dreams and memories can nurture us only if we build a proper nest where they feel welcome. We need a place to collapse under the weight of grief when it gets too great—a place to gaze at the moon-shadows playing across the walls, and—when nights are especially long—to watch the slow dawning of the new day. It took me fifty-something years, three degrees, two marriages, three children, and skirmishes with any number of roofers and ceiling-guys and landscape architects to finally hear this truth.

Home-improvement is an overwhelming thing, but I'm beginning to get the idea. Curb appeal will be nice in its time. But the point here is to build a sanctuary—a place where loved ones share stories and meals, where art and music can be enjoyed—a place where souls can rest and regroup when the press of the world seems too great. A place, at last, for a midlife woman to create a watercolor room in which to house her dreams.

I can't wait to see those walls take shape. I can't wait to rest and imagine there, letting my thoughts unfold. And I can't wait to burst through those French doors, into the waiting dawn.

Questions for Reflection:

1. Do you have a retreat place in your house? A private corner with a meditation chair? A room decorated with pleasing colors and lush green plants? A garden spot surrounded by beauty? Imagine your ideal spot. You may want to gather pictures and ideas out of magazines and put them in your journal.

*Daphne Stevens*

2. As you go about your shopping, errands, or travels, pick up things that support your need for contemplation and retreat—pillows, artwork, books you long to read, CDs of your favorite music. Put them in your own "watercolor bedroom—" or store them in a safe place as you create your home retreat.

# Chapter 3: Feeding the Muse

How do you cope with stress? It's a question I hear often in my role as a therapist.

The truth is that some days I do well to just put one foot in front of the other. The tedium of paying the bills, the relentlessness of grief, the press of a culture that devalues the inner life, the tension between my longing to relieve suffering and my desire to simply escape—it all seems too much. A kind of plodding discipline overtakes me. When duty overshadows the joy of life, resentment is never far behind.

But on grace-filled days, I remember that pain can be a manifestation of unclaimed creative gifts. It is a truth the culture often overlooks, and it is true of all of us: Those places where we ignore our creativity tend to show up in the form of symptoms.

Nurturing your creativity means attending to things that bring joy for their own sake. Tending a garden. Doing needlepoint. Creating a special meal. Dancing to Motown music. Writing in a journal. Telling someone your dreams. My five-year-old grandson knows how to do it when he plays in the sandbox for hours on end, building communities and playing out dramas with his collection of tiny figurines. This process of entering into the imaginal world—of using our bodies and our imaginations in unexpected ways— is magic. It's healing. It's restorative.

Last New Year's Eve, a small group my friends gathered together. After an evening of lamenting the traumas that the autumn had brought, we began to ask ourselves some questions: What do we want to let go of as we end this year? What do we want to invite into our lives as we enter into the next phase? We wrote down those things we most wanted to relinquish, and as midnight approached, we threw them with abandon into the fire. Anxiety, fear, guilt, the urge to control things we couldn't control—all went up in flames. Then we offered one another images of things we want to invite into our lives: Balance, abundant life, joy, spontaneity, and a love of truth for its own sake came into the room as poetic visions we enacted for one another right there on the spot.

Maybe all of us will be just as neurotic this year as we were in the past—but around the fire on New Year's Eve, we entered into creative space together. We will be fortified for the challenges of the coming year, having entered into the truer-than-true fantasy that, even in the face of searing grief, life doesn't have to be deadly serious all the time.

It's a fantasy that, for me, always signals the return of emotional and spiritual wellness— no matter how daunting the challenges may be.

Questions for Reflection:

1. What are the traits or issues in yourself that you'd like to relinquish as you enter into the next phase of your life? Write them down on a piece of paper.

2. Ask yourself the question, "What has living with each of these things taught me about myself? Am I ready to claim that lesson as my own?"

3. Write down any wisdom that comes to you, and appreciate yourself for the grace to discern the message built into the symptom or difficulty.

4. Alone or with a group of friends, create a ritual to let go of the things you are ready to relinquish.

# Chapter 4: Creating a Vision

What do you want to be when you grow up?

"I want to be a doctor." "I want to be a mommy." "I want to be an astronaut and go to Mars." Ask any small child in your life, and see how she warms to the question: Children are visionaries by nature.

In young adulthood, our visions sharpen into goals. "I want to go to this college or that." "I want to join the Peace Corps for a year." "I want to find the right person and start a family." Our achievements are marked with grades, awards, and ceremonies.

As we transition into midlife, our lenses soften into a visionary mode. Where do you want to be in six months? In a year? In five years? In ten? The answers require the achievement of goals—but without vision, the goals become empty exercises, more hoops to jump through in a time of life when most of us are tired of achievement for achievement's sake.

If I ask you about your goals, you might say, "I want to build up enough money in my retirement plan to be able to be comfortable and free." If I ask you about your vision, I am asking, "What does 'comfortable' look like/feel like/smell like to you? What are your images of comfort?" And "What does 'freedom' mean? Freedom from anxiety? Freedom to work at your own pace to pursue old passions or a new career? Freedom to travel?"

People who are full of goals but short on visions say things like, "I have so much to be thankful for—a good job, nice house, great children, etc. But it all feels so empty. Where do I fit into my own life?" People who are full of visions but short on goals say, "How do I get from here to there?" They are deluged with big ideas and schemes that dissipate, only to be replaced with other big ideas that never seem to materialize. They tend to feel like victims.

Midlife is a time rich with visions. The goals we have met in our younger years—the skills we have built, the wisdom we have earned, the investments we have made—free us to imagine a life we can love.

Visions come from many sources. Childhood yearnings are one rich source. Night-time dreams are another. Recurrent fantasies that begin with things like, "If I had enough money (or time) I would. . ." are signs that a vision is trying to claim you.

Creating a vision is a little like falling in love. You start with an image: "This looks like the woman/man for me." You begin to get focused on developing that relationship. Your other pursuits begin to take second place, and you find yourself organizing your life around being with your beloved. If the love affair is viable, your beloved meets you more than halfway. Nothing will be right until you can be together. Both you and your partner experience the relationship as a great miracle, and details of life are ordered around the mystery of that connection. You are, in essence, claimed by love.

A vision claims us, just like love does. It takes on a life of its own. "I'd like to live in a house on the lake" materializes in the form of a house plan or a piece of land. We begin to set goals to live into that vision. We may be blocked at every turn, but we are now on a hero's quest. The house (or the love, or the career, or the book we want to write) has claimed us as its own.

My friend Heather is building a house. After thirty years of marriage devoted to the running of a household, the support of a husband's career, and the raising of five children, she finds herself alone. She is living every woman's nightmare—bereft of a spouse and without education or resume.

But Heather has been claimed by a vision. She doesn't have a lot of fancy diplomas on her wall to prove her genius. She simply has a gift for being resourceful and persistent, for being a good neighbor, for creating beauty around her, and for bringing people together.

Heather doesn't linger long in her grief—I suspect there will be layers of that to uncover in time—but she has asked herself some crucial questions. "What have I always dreamed about? How would I truly like to live?" After years of moving from place to place to promote her husband's career, Heather longs for a house of her own.

Heather has used her gifts for years in the service of others, and now she is using them in the service of her own vision. Every vision calls forth "angels"— folks who show up with a special skill or a gift or a word of encouragement. An architect has volunteered his services. A forester has delivered a bundle of dogwoods to plant around the site. A demolished house has provided windows and doors and a hot water heater and kitchen cabinets. A circle of women gathered together recently to consecrate the

*Watercolor Bedroom*

land where the house will be built. Some of Heather's angels have come to help her haul stones for the fireplace that will be the center of her small home in the woods. "This will be the house that women built," she proclaims.

Every goal along the way to claiming a vision can seem like a major obstacle. Hauling windows and hot water heaters and kitchen cabinets and stones. Getting building permits and finding financing. Heather isn't through it all yet. But she is driven by her vision. She anticipates throwing a party for her angels when the house becomes a reality. What she sometimes forgets is that her angels are already blessed, simply for having been a part of Heather's unfolding vision.

Like neglected loves, visions move into the background if we don't give them their due. While we can't force them to re-enter our lives, we can create hospitable space and invite them to speak. We can honor them in small daily ways, or in huge courageous steps like Heather has. Either way, we change the course of our lives.

With each step, we claim our destiny. With each step, we bless the lives of others.

Questions for Reflection:
1. In your journal, complete the following sentences:
   When I was little, I wanted to be _____.
   Some things that I love to do are _____.
   A day (or a week) in my ideal life would be _____.

2. What do these sentences tell you about your vision? What goals are you pursuing to make that vision a reality?

# Chapter 5: Snakes and Angels

"I don't mean to whine," a woman recently lamented, "but living into a vision isn't as easy as you make it sound. I'm fully committed to getting my degree, and ever since I went back to school I've felt I'm on a mission. But I've never been so tired."

She has reason to be tired. She is working full time and caring for an ailing mother. Her college kids frequently show up on weekends. Her husband travels, leaving her to run the household by herself. But none of these problems seem to be the source of her exhaustion.

"All I hear are complaints. My boss wants me to stay late when she knows I have to go straight to class. My mother says I don't visit her enough in the nursing home, even though I go three times a week. My children complain about too much take-out food on weekends. My husband thinks school just may be too much for me to take on. Where are these Angels you talk about?"

We had talked at length about Angels, but I had forgotten to mention Snakes.

When we are living into a vision, Snakes show up. They are far less welcome and pleasant than Angels, but they are just as crucial. Some folks might say that Snakes appear to test our determination, to shape our character or the like. I don't know about that. I just know they show up.

In the Garden of Eden, the Snake tempted Eve to eat the fruit of the Tree of Knowledge. Being weak and womanly, she listened to the Snake, and then tempted her mate, who (being weak and manly) listened to her. Snakes (and women) have gotten a bad rap ever since.

In postmodern times, Snakes distract us from the fruits of the trees that might lead us further into living our vision. "Be careful," is their universal chorus. "Are you sure you're Good Enough?"

Snakes show up early in most of our lives. They take the form of teachers who thwart our creativity with red-penciled admonitions condemning grammatical transgressions that sully our first attempt at poetry. They appear as parents who say things like, "You're just like your father (or aunt or brother). He was never any good at math." They show up as god-parents who say, "You don't mean that!" when we express passionate feelings about anything at all. By the time we are grown up, most of us have been well trained to confuse our own voices with the echoes of the Snake voices reverberating in our heads.

For the past fifty years psychotherapy has focused on the idea that if you can separate a person from her Snakes, she will be healthy and free. Having traveled that road as a therapist and as a client, I've come to the conclusion that Snakes are grossly under-rated. Snakes, in fact, are powerful medicine.

When we are creating a midlife vision, Snakes show up in myriad ways. They say things like "You can't afford to do this!" and "How can you take time away from your family?" And (more benevolently) "Don't you think you're in just a little over your head? After all, you're 45 (or 35 or 60) years old."

Some Snakes can be even snakier. They show up as spouses or lovers who betray you. They make a cameo appearance as a jealous colleague who wreaks havoc on your life by stealing your ideas or setting you up to look bad with your boss. We want to overlook them. Nobody could be that mean, we tell ourselves. I must be too sensitive.

But, as J.D. Salinger once said, "just because you're paranoid doesn't mean they're not out to get you." And when you're living into a vision, you're in trouble if you're not prepared to reckon with Snakes.

Native Americans had a deep respect for Snakes. Not having heard about Adam and Eve, they knew that all animals had wisdom and power. Living into a vision meant learning about every animal that crossed your path. When you dreamed a dream about a deer, or when a rabbit scampered across the meadow in the twilight, you would go to a sacred teepee where the elders were holding counsel. You'd ask questions like, "What does this creature have to say to me about living my vision?"

Snakes were said to bestow special gifts. Because they moved easily back and forth between the under-world and the upper-world, they were thought to possess supernatural powers. Because they regularly shed their skin, they carried the capacity for healing and regeneration. A person who had survived the bite of a poisonous snake was believed to have visited the Other World, and therefore to hold shamanic powers.

The truth is that most of us have been bitten by poisonous snakes, and when one shows up in the midst of our vision, it can mean we are particularly blessed. But when we talk about our Snakes to others, we hear things like, "You poor thing!" Therapists and friends and new lovers can be the worst people to turn to when we have a bad case of snake-bite. They may give us empathy instead of asking the central question, "What is the thing you have learned about yourself from this wound?"

So what use *are* Snakes when we're living into a vision? I want to tell you a secret.

In the blink of an eye a Snake can turn into an Angel. And in another blink, an Angel can turn into a Snake.

Does this mean they are interchangeable? No. An Angel is still an Angel and a Snake is still a Snake, and if you get them confused, you are worse than naïve. You betray your vision when you entrust yourself to a Snake. You can pay for it with years of wasted effort.

Learning from a Snake is a delicate business—but it is the only way to escape a kind of living death. In the willingness to learn, a miracle can take place.

If, when we are snake-bit, we ask ourselves the question, "What is the lesson?" the Snake can be transformed.

A transformed Snake may be the unfaithful lover who prompts us to ask ourselves, "How did I happen to entrust myself to him?" A transformed Snake may be the plagiarizing colleague who challenges us to wonder, "How was she able to see my idea as something valuable, when I didn't see it myself?"

It's miserable recovering from Snake-bite. Sometimes it takes years. But sometimes it only takes a moment of stepping outside the cozy comfort of empathic friends, and into the courage to look at ourselves and the world with the moral toughness of snake-eyes.

Don't get me wrong. Empathic presence can give us a nest in which to garner our strength and take the next steps toward living into our vision. Angels can give us hope. But when we insist on Angels to the exclusion of Snakes, we cheat ourselves. We betray our vision. We write imaginary happy endings that deprive us of the lessons gleaned from weathering disappointment and pain.

Questions for Reflection:

1. Who are the "Snakes" that have inhabited your world? Think about any scenario that comes to mind: an abusive parent, an unfaithful spouse, a friend who betrayed your confidence, a difficult boss. List them in your journal.

2. Now, consider yourself as you reflect on each person. To what extent do you feel victimized by this person or situation? You might mark a "V" beside each name that still elicits pain for you.

3. Consider the possibility that you are still feeling wounded because there is a gift you have failed to claim from your experience with this person—perhaps a realization that you reveal yourself too easily or that you trust too readily. How can you begin to protect yourself when faced with these "problem" people?

4. If there are "Snakes" you can now name as "Angels," give thanks for your wisdom as well as for those lessons. Wish those people well and release them. They have given you a gift.

## Chapter 6: Demeter's Daughter

I'm always curious when my own writing talks back to me.

A recent journal entry quizzed me as I took my morning walk. "You said in your younger days you prayed a lot for people. Did you mean that praying for people is a function of immaturity or youthful idealism?"

Of course not. Today I pray even more. The difference is that, embedded in the prayers of my youth was the assumption that I knew something. Now I know I know nothing.

It's embarrassing to admit how much I prayed for outcome. "God—help this person to get better. Or to realize this or that. Or to heal. Or to find You." Or any of a number of prayers attached to various outcomes that assumed I knew what "better" or "this or that" or "heal" or even "You" meant. My prayers these days are more of the "thank you- thank you- thank you-thank you" genre and the "Thy will be done-Thy will be done-Thy will be done" variety. I sense the prayers in the rhythm of my footsteps as I walk, in my out-breath as I wait for sleep to come at night, in the sound of my husband's heartbeat as I lie against his chest in the wee hours of the morning. I feel them in the pulse of life that reverberates through our two bodies and in the sense of peace that engulfs me when I listen to summer crickets singing outside my window.

I am dumb. I do not know what to pray for. I am grateful for that dumbness.

*Watercolor Bedroom*

This dumbness did not come easily to me. It came after long hard years of being convinced that I could or should have answers.

In my youth, I followed the rules. I married a man for what I thought were the right reasons. I raised a child by the books. And I painstaking learned that many of the rules of my sophomoric twenties were ultimately terribly wrong— and that my beautiful golden-haired child would defy everything I thought I knew about motherhood, unconditional love, and what children need.

The ancient Greeks told a story. Persephone, adored by her mother Demeter, was abducted by Hades and swooped into the Underworld. Demeter was devastated by her daughter's disappearance. As do grieving mothers everywhere, Demeter refused to eat or drink; she appealed to god after god for the whereabouts of her daughter, but no one would tell her the truth. Finally, she appealed to the Sun, who told her the terrible story: Persephone was beneath the earth living among the shadowy dead.

Demeter fell into an even deeper grief. She left her station as a goddess and lived among mortals, disguised as a peasant nursemaid to the infant son of a village family. By day she fed him sweet ambrosia, and by night she laid him in the heart of the fire's red-hot coals so that he could attain eternal youth.

But the baby's mother became uneasy. Walking in on Demeter in the middle of the night, she gasped in horror to see her child being laid in the fire. Demeter rose up to her full height as a goddess, threw off her peasant-woman disguise, and filled the room with her radiance. The household was amazed and immediately set about the work of building

Demeter a temple. When it was finished, Demeter withdrew into it, wasting away and grieving for her daughter.

Now Demeter was also the goddess of the grain, and while she languished, no crops would grow. It seemed as if the earth's people would die of famine. The gods appealed to Demeter one by one, but she refused to give energy to the earth until she could see her daughter. Hermes, the messenger-god, was finally sent into the underworld to appeal to Hades to return his bride to her mother.

Persephone, meanwhile, had greatly missed her mother. Hades reluctantly released her—but he asked her to eat a pomegranate seed before she left, knowing that if she did so she would have to return to him.

Well, we can imagine the grand reunion that took place. Mother and daughter talked all day about what had happened to them both. Demeter was grieved to hear about the pomegranate seed, knowing that Persephone now belonged to the Underworld—indeed, was its Queen there—and would have to return there for part of each year. This is how the ancient Greeks explained the season of winter.

We have fancier ways of understanding the winter season in our culture, but I sure understand Demeter. My daughter is a Persephone girl. She dropped out of my sight into the underworld when she was a teenager. Like Demeter, I appealed to all the gods—the teachers, the tutors, the therapists, the doctors—those who were supposed to know—and no one could tell me her whereabouts.

I'm no divine being, but I did the Demeter thing. I refused to take nourishment, thinking that if I did so long enough my daughter would be restored to me. I nurtured other people's children as best I knew how. I continued to appeal to the experts. And after years and years I began to throw off my disguise and assume my full stature as a (somewhat flawed) goddess. When I began to show up in my own life, the gods intervened—and my daughter ever so slowly began to be restored to me.

This is what I have learned. My daughter has a serious, chronic illness. It is not her fault. It is not my fault. Her illness has compromised her ability to learn some important skills and lessons. She has some remedial work to do—but then, so do I. Her illness means that ordinary things—getting up in the mornings some days, for example—are supreme expressions of courage. Her illness means that controlling her impulses and staying focused and finishing tasks are sometimes gargantuan acts of will.

But I've learned more. I've been freed from the cause-and-effect "Follow the rules/Get your reward" myth that destined me to eternal disillusionment and disappointment and bitterness. I've learned that I almost never get what I deserve—and I've learned to thank God for that.

The Greeks don't tell us the end of the story—what happened to Demeter in subsequent winters. I know my own landscape can look pretty bleak when my daughter is feeling lost. But I like to imagine Demeter awakening on a winter's day feeling weary of the taste of her own grief. "There's nothing to be done here for now," she might have sighed, getting up and washing her face, "It's the darkest day of the year." So she might have created a feast and summoned her friends—and as the night fell, she might have lit candles to defy the darkness. I like to imagine that in that darkness, the first winter holiday party was born.

And I like to imagine that the singing and the laughter and the revelry of that party might have been bright enough even to gladden the heart of Persephone—the Queen of the Underworld—as she waited in her underground lair for the inevitable coming of Spring.

Questions for Reflection:

1. Where are the places in your life where you have known (or continue to know) disappointment, anxiety, fear, and frustration about someone you deeply love? List those people in your journal.

2. Assume for a moment that you have done everything possible to remedy the situation.

3. Now, think about your role in that person's life—not your fantasy of yourself as a hero, or the culture's myth that "If you love somebody enough, you can save them." You'll probably find that your role right now in that loved one's life is pretty limited—that you are a minor player in the life they are creating.

4. Consider taking a vacation from guilt and anxiety for awhile. It may be a weekend away with your spouse. It may be a regular meeting with a support group. It may be a 12-step program, or it may be in the simple act of saying to your loved one, "I love you. I don't know how to solve these problems—and for now I need a recess. I trust your ability to begin to come up with your own solutions."

5. Set a boundary—a few weeks without contact, or a certain hour after which you don't discuss problems at night.

6. Recruit a few friends to support you in your resolve to avoid perpetuating the problem or treating your loved one like an invalid. Notice how you feel in a few weeks or months.

# Chapter 7: Dream-Tending

Today was a cold and blustery Sunday. As I settled by the fire with my coffee and newspaper, a young friend called. "Do you have time to listen to a dream I had last night? "Sure," I replied, ready for a cozy telephone chat. But she was much more eager. "I'll be over in 20 minutes." I cast my newspaper aside without a second thought, and began to prepare more coffee. I sensed that it was going to be a lively morning.

Why do I listen for dreams so intently? It's because the lives of dreamers have brought me a wisdom too deep for words. Dreams provide one of the few psychic inroads not blocked by a "sound-bite" culture that overloads us with information and stifles the imagination. I am always ready to listen.

When we sleep, the images of the night visit us. They tell us something about the loamy inner life of the psyche. They signal us about a layer of reality too often lost in the day-world. They remind us of the there-then-gone moments of intuition or fantasy or poetry that get submerged in the deluge of appointments and schedules.

When we see ourselves only as the world defines us, we neglect vital aspects of our psychic lives. We define ourselves only as mother or wife, as teacher or doctor, as liberal or conservative. We forget the ways that we might want to play, to create, to celebrate, to mourn. We ignore those incarnations of the Divine that come to remind us that we all share in the collective genius (and the collective darkness) of humankind.

When we slow down enough to listen to our dreams, we know more about the ways we are interconnected with the whole of the human community. We remember the ways that the Divine and the human dance within us, and we more consciously join in that dance.

Midlife is a time for listening to dreams. As we listen, we connect with the rich shadowy aspects of Self that have gotten lost in the rush of a life dominated by the dictates of the Ego. We are free to accept the gifts nestled within, and we become more accepting toward ourselves and others.

I keep my dreams in a journal. I find that by writing them down, I give them their due and start the day in a self-reflective way that is closely akin to prayer. I find that dreams will often speak in unexpected ways when I go back to them at a later phase of my life. It's as though my soul's depths know something that my ego isn't yet ready to take in. I often understand a dream on a number of different levels as I continue my life's journey. In that way, the dreams continue to bless and inform me—a great source of comfort and wisdom and strength.

Archetypal psychologist Stephen Aizenstat refers to this listening as "tending." Through tending our dreams, we stay curious about them. We get to know them as we might get acquainted with an unexpected visitor in our home. We value their mystery enough to create rituals to cultivate them and to mine their meaning. We share them with a friend.

*Daphne Stevens*

In dream-tending, we come home to ourselves and to the larger human family.

Have you ever shared a dream with someone who really listened, without feeling closer to that person? Dreams provide most of us with our purest encounter with our own creativity—and, when we share them, they offer us our purest experience of human affinity. Have you noticed the eyes of a child as she recounts a vivid dream to an interested grownup? I think about that—and I wonder what it might be like if children in school were encouraged to talk about their dreams— to draw them, to write them, to re-enact them in play. What might be the gifts received by a community devoted to encouraging its children to revel in their own imaginations and to trust their inner visions? What do we lose by discounting that treasure—by dismissing dreams out of hand?

I sat at noon today with my young friend in front of the dying embers, gazing into my empty coffee cup. The room was resonant with the voices of dream figures that had visited us, and my friend was radiant in the morning sun. As I smiled into her warm brown eyes, I remembered Jungian writer Marie-Louise Von Franz's description of dreamers. She described the dreamer as "insignificant individual who holds the thread in the palm of her unknowing hand."

My sense is that my young friend indeed holds that thread, and that it is leading her somewhere precious and life-giving.

*Watercolor Bedroom*

Questions for Reflection:

1. What is the first dream you remember, as a child or a young adult? Jot it down and reflect on it. How do you see the images or themes of the dream lived out as you think about your life's unfolding story?

2. Keep a dream journal for the next week. For seven days, go to bed asking the Divine presence to make your dreams manifest to you. In the morning, allow time to write down anything that comes—a snippet, an image, even a feeling. Often these dream fragments are profound in their gifts.

3. Set aside time with a trusted friend, a spiritual director, or a therapist who is attuned to dreams. Devote that time to "mining" your dreams for the week—attending to the images, listening to the voices, and asking the question, "What do these dreams want?"

4. Create a response to a dream—any response. An art project or a walk in the woods or a visit to a museum, in honor of a dream, will heighten the dream's power to bless your life.

# Chapter 8: Changing Careers

I've been thinking a lot about this midlife task of letting go. Sometimes it means forgiving other people, and sometimes it means letting go of something in ourselves.

Take me, for example. After more years than I want to admit, I have decided to change careers. I won't be giving up my psychotherapy practice, nor will I stop coaching people toward their dreams. But I've decided to give up worrying.

I don't take this step lightly. In fact, I've talked to some of the smartest people I know about it, and I've gotten some admonitions.

"Are you sure you want to give up worrying?" my husband asks, his brow furrowed. "You're always talking about the archetype of the Worrier-Woman. It seems so important to you." "That's *Warrior*-Woman," I tell him. But, in truth, I've had Worriers confused with Warriors for far too long.

I come from a long line of worriers. In my family it's what we do to show that we care. My mother was the champion worrier. "You sound stopped up. Are you coming down with something?" was her standard way of greeting me. My father is a close runner-up. "You look exhausted. Are you working too hard?" are his code-words for "I'm proud of you." My brothers and my aunt regularly call me up just to remind me of things to worry about. I have to admit that I feel a little guilty about giving up the family business, but I have myself to think about. I also have to look ahead and set a good example for my children. I mean, when I'm old and sick, do I want a bunch of sleep-deprived hand-wringers hanging around my bed? No. I want them fresh and well-rested. I also want them to be interesting. I want them to be energized so they can pamper me in the way in which I plan to become accustomed.

My friend Tina, another Worrier-turned-Warrior, cautions me about making a big career change too fast. "Don't be hasty," she suggests. "There must be some market value in being an expert, high-detail worrier—not just an ordinary one, but a really talented one—one who could investigate all the nooks and crannies of possible misfortunes. Clients could be out playing bridge or shopping while YOU charge them big bucks to have Kafka-esque worries in their stead. You could give discounts for less bizarre worries like whether a meteorite will hit the earth in their lifetime. You'd have to charge more to come up with worries they never even considered—like what if their relative changed his name to Gregor Samsa and turned into a roach."

"Very funny," I say to Tina. "I spent the first part of my life getting advanced degrees to become a therapist. I was convinced at the time that I was making meaning out of my life and helping people. But now I see that I was getting credentialed to hire out as a professional worrier. The benefits are lousy, and the pay isn't great. There has to be another way to make a living."

The deliberations were lengthy, but the actual decision to give up worrying came in a flash. I had just received one of those phone calls unique to midlife. I don't remember the details just now, but you probably know the story: An elderly relative is in a crisis in the nursing home, or a young adult child is in a predicament on the job, or a grandchild has an ear infection. I was already exhausted from a hard day's work, and, in a blaze of insight about why they call us the "sandwich generation," I went into a panic. This isn't ever going to get any better, I moaned to myself. I wrapped up in the fetal position in a full-blown and well-earned anxiety attack for almost an hour, just waiting for someone to die or the world to go away.

Nobody died, and nothing went away, but something unexpected happened. As I lay there with my heart pounding, preparing to engage in a Worrying Marathon, I found myself hovering over my body. Oh, great, I thought. What now? A Near-Death Experience or a psychotic episode, on top of everything else? I cautiously opened one eye, curious to see what would happen next.

As I hovered over my body, watching myself curled up on the bed, I suddenly had a sanity attack. "Is this worrying helping anybody?" I found myself asking. (NO, I had to admit from under the covers.) "Is this worrying helping me to become a better person?" (NO, I sniffed, clutching my pillow even harder.) "Is this worrying making the world a better place?" (NO.) "Have I EVER really solved a problem or helped another person or resolved any of my own suffering by worrying?" (NO. NO. NO.) "Oh."

The room got really quiet. I felt my body relax.

I somewhat begrudgingly un-clutched my pillow. "Okay," I said to my husband. "I'm through. Take me to the movies." A good melodrama is usually helpful in releasing me from the grip of my own troubles. I figured that the phone call-induced crisis could wait for a couple of hours. As it turned out, the caller managed to work out the problem without my help, and my husband and I had a nice evening out.

Over the weeks since that sanity attack, I've had to get downright pushy about anxiety. I see it as the enemy; if I let it in, it whispers nasty lies to me. "You have to suffer to be of service," it might say to me in certain moods. Or, "You have to earn your place on the planet." Or—this is my favorite one—"What kind of a Mother are you anyway, just having a good time, when your children aren't fully self-actualized and settled and happy?"

They are old lies—I've heard them for a long time—but now I mean business about banishing them. I might dismiss them by telling a difficult truth to someone I care about. I might send them away with physical exercise. I've become a great fan of kick-boxing—a powerful weapon in the war against anxiety demons. And I lift weights, pushing away worries (and osteoporosis) with every vigorous exhalation. Lamaze, I'm finding, was a great training ground for breathing through the birthing pains of moving through midlife neurosis. And I'm feeling better and better.

Don't get me wrong. I'm still cautious about this career change of mine. I'm not making any rash irreversible decisions. I figure if the sky in fact begins to fall just because I'm not trying to hold it up, I can always go back to worrying.

But for now—just for today—I'm giving it up.

Questions for Reflection:

1. What are the things that worry you the most? Jot down a quick list in your journal.

2. Go down the list. Which items do you actually have control over? Which situations will get better by your staying anxious?

3. Now, jot down an "action list"—things to do to dispel anxiety when you are tempted to worry about things you can't change. Exercising, meditating, going to the movies, pulling weeds in the garden—think of all the options you can.

4. Keep both lists with you this week. When you're tempted by an item on your Worry List, go to your Action List and get moving. Notice any changes in your feelings.

# Chapter 9: Ash Wednesday

Ash Wednesday. I nestle comfortably into the pew between my husband and my daughter to be reminded of the frailty of my physical being and the brevity of my stay here on earth. I draw solace from words that have been prayed for centuries, receiving the Imposition of the Ashes and hearing the ancient mantra, "From dust you came and to dust you shall return."

I remember when I used to hear that somber liturgy as the Voice of Doom, an ominous warning of the sureness of death. At this phase of my life I begin to hear it as one of life's loving promises: The suffering, the cruelty, the anxiety here on earth, is only temporary. "Dust to Dust" is a parenthetical phrase, reminding me of the ever-present mystery of life beyond what we know.

My daughter— so brave, so free, so grown-up these days—holds my hand throughout the service. We silently light a prayer candle for a favorite aunt who is dying. She is never far from our minds.

I am joyful in this body of mine, even as I draw strange comfort from its finitude. I work out hard at the gym, often dripping with sweat by the time I am finished, and then I swim hard steady laps for an hour. The words of the liturgy sing through the workout: "This fragile earth, our island home." It's how I think of my body these days. It's a pleasure to be alive.

*Daphne Stevens*

  The same incongruity is reflected in the turn of the season this year. In an early morning walk this week, I noticed the tender beginnings of buds on the crepe myrtle trees lining the sidewalk of Ridge Avenue. A bird's nest—was it from last year or this year?—was starkly visible against the gray streaks of dawn. The cold-weather camellia blossoms still clung to the bushes that line the other side of my path. Dark to dawn. Winter to spring. Ashes to ashes. Dust to dust. The songs of the season call me into work, into prayer, into rest.

  In this culture, we live in a world of perpetual illusions of triumph, and Lent is much under-rated. Resurrection and victory are our themes. It is valiant, perhaps, to live with such pluck—to pretend that the Dark Night of the Soul is an avoidable malady, a blip on the screen of continuous optimism. But we deprive our souls of good nourishment, I'm afraid, by our insistence on buoyancy and brightness.

  Spring heralds its coming, there's no doubt of that; bird-songs call out among the multicolored blossoms. "It's here!" they seem to say. "Come out and play! Rejoice, oh sad, tired humanity! Shed your winter clothes and come barefoot onto the greening lawn of life."

  Yet the dark days of Lent attune my eyes to subtle hues in the kaleidoscope of life's changes. I watch for the slivers of dreams that dance on the edge of my consciousness, savoring the presence of mysteries that have not yet revealed their secrets. I suspend the anticipation of Easter colors to linger a little longer in the land of purple-toned penitence. I want to stay and be nourished here awhile, before spring calls me into its glorious exuberance.

Questions for Reflection:

1. How do you experience paradox in your life—the richness of grief or the melancholy inherent in joyous celebration?

2. Some families save a place at the table for the "Christ guest"—the unexpected visitor who might show up for holiday dinners. Others leave the chair of a departed loved one empty to recognize his or her absence. How do you acknowledge the presence of loved ones no longer with you?

3. When did you experience the most vivid celebration of spring? Perhaps it was the year you married, the year you were pregnant, or when you embarked on a special adventure. Write a paragraph in your journal remembering that younger, idealistic, naïve self.

4. Write a love letter to your body. Tell your body what you appreciate about how it serves you—its strengths, its reminders of both your mortality and your preciousness. And make a promise to your body, too. Make a specific note about how you plan to cherish your physical being through this spring and summer season.

# Chapter 10: A Pink Blanket of Love

The term "minor surgery" is an oxymoron. We use it to refer to someone else's medical procedure—never our own. When we are placed under general anesthesia for the purpose of being cut, probed, excised, or explored, it's going to be a major event.

I am home this week recovering from such an event. I have "done well," as they say. My recuperation has surpassed all expectations—particularly my own. I am almost enjoying this visit into quasi-invalidism—and I am learning a lot.

I was blessed in preparing for this. In researching options for easing my road to recovery, I discovered a book called *Prepare for Surgery, Heal Faster* by Peggy Huddleston. Peggy suggests that by following five simple steps—regular relaxation, visualization of healing, recruiting friends to pray for you during surgery, asking that your doctor make positive "healing statements" while you are under the anesthesia, and meeting your anesthesiologist ahead of time—you can dramatically reduce your level of post-operative discomfort, speed your healing, and increase your sense of well being.

Going under general anesthesia, after all, is the closest most of us come (in the course of this life) to being dead. Having our bodies invaded by strangers is a psychic and physical violation, no matter how optimistic we may feel about the benefits of the procedure. Peggy Huddleston understands this profoundly.

*Watercolor Bedroom*

    I was surprised one evening by a phone message from Peggy. "I was concerned about whether you received the book and the tape in ample time for your surgery," she said. "I realized your order had gone out a couple of days after it was due, and wanted to make sure you had the materials in time." Well, I had ordered the materials in plenty of time—my surgery wasn't scheduled for another five weeks—but I marveled at her concern. After all, she knew nothing about me except the ordering information I had left on her web site. I didn't respond to the phone message, but I thanked the Universe for people like Peggy, and felt more encouraged in preparing for my adventure.

    As I read into the book, I began to get energized. My sense of dread—the anticipation of being a passive-if-willing "victim"—began to shift into a realization that I could be an active agent in my own healing. As I practiced listening to Peggy's relaxation tapes, I began to see the surgery as an event—almost an athletic event, if you will—for which I could condition myself, psychically and physically. My daily walks became more vigorous. I devoted more attention to nutrition, savoring every meal as a source of profound nurturing. I realized that I hadn't paid such loving attention to my body since the days of pregnancy years ago. Just as those days were devoted to birthing new life, this preparation time was becoming dedicated to birthing myself—my older, wiser, second-half-of-life self.

    But Peggy surprised me yet again. About a week before the surgery date, she called me on a Saturday night. "I'm doing a workshop here in Cambridge," she said. One of my trainees would like to offer you an hour by phone tomorrow morning to help you prepare more fully." I agreed readily. During the course of my chat with Peggy, I shared my experiences supporting my own clients through medical challenges. I expressed excitement about the prospect of sharing her book with others—and I thanked her for her interest in my own healing process.

The next morning, I spoke with Peggy's student, a young woman named Eden St. James, who is a recent graduate of Barbara Brennan's world-renowned school of energy healing. Eden's new degree was of particular interest to me; I am fortunate to have worked for several years with Pamela Englebert, a Brennan graduate who practices energy healing in my home town. I told Eden of my work with Pamela; I had, in fact, met with Pamela just a few days earlier for an energy healing session.

Eden began the phone session by inviting me to share my concerns. I discovered that, despite all my good intentions, I was predicting less than the best for myself. "I'll be under the anesthesia for three hours," I said. "That's what you've been *told*," Eden gently clarified. I realized—yes—it could be less extensive than that: The surgeon can only go on her experience, not on what she knows about my body or my level of readiness, so why should I assume the worst? "I've been told the pain will be awful," I lamented. "It could be that you'll be quite comfortable," Eden replied. Well, that was true, too. I had heard from other people about their experiences—but other people aren't me. In trying to achieve some measure of control over my own anxiety by embracing a worst-case-scenario, I had managed to make myself more anxious.

One by one, I named my worries. Then Eden asked me an important question. "If everything goes ideally, what will you be saying to yourself right after the surgery?"

I hesitated. "I'll be saying, 'I'm not in much pain.'"

Again, Eden was gentle. What about: "I'm comfortable?"

Well, based on what I had been told, it seemed a lot to ask. But I decided to go with the moment.

"Okay. 'I'm comfortable.'" It felt like I wasn't giving the Pain-and-Suffering Gods their due, but why not go for it? If I woke up in agony, I could always say, "I give up! The Pain Gods won!" with no loss of face. I am, after all, only human.

The next part of the session was a lovely hypnotic induction. Eden eased me into a deep state of relaxation, and then she walked me through each step of the process—the pre-op, the slide into unconsciousness, the waking-up in a state of ease and comfort, the two weeks' recovery at home—and then imagining the way I wanted to feel several months after the surgery. I envisioned myself fully recovered, healthy and vibrant, doing the things I love. I saw myself biking with my husband on a crisp autumn day. I saw myself in the classroom and the consulting room, fully confident and present, filled with a sense of vitality. I saw myself snuggling with my grandsons, baking Christmas cookies, making love with my husband. In my vision, I enjoyed my body in a way I've never felt before—middle-aged, yes, and fit and filled with the joy of life.

The vision held me in its arms. I'm at home recovering, now, and marveling at what I've learned. I've learned that expectations have everything to do with experience. I've found that walking through this with a loving, respectful, non-anxious circle of friends has transformed a potential trauma into an opportunity to feel God's love on a physical level I have never quite known before.

I'm also humbled by my own good fortune. It helps that I am blessed with excellent health. It's been a great boon to find my physician and anesthesiologist to be eager partners in my preparation process. A small circle of friends has supported me, keeping me supplied with chicken soup and flowers and books and cards. And it doesn't hurt that I am companioned by a husband who has basically put his work on hold in order to devote himself to plying me with freshly juiced vegetable and fruit concoctions and back-rubs and jokes and sympathy, depending on my whim. Yes, I am fully blessed.

But I have learned even more. Peggy suggests that, when you prepare for surgery, you don't just ask your friends to pray for you in a generic way. She suggests that you ask them to imagine you wrapped in a blanket of love. You envision the color and the kind of blanket you want to enfold you; the idea is that, when the senses and imagination are engaged, prayer becomes a more palpable experience, both for the pray-er and for the pray-ee. My blanket is pink and velvety-soft, the way I imagined the insides of the rosebuds in my wedding bouquet some years ago.

I'm discovering that life is filled with opportunities for learning and deepening. Fear and anxiety and suffering are everywhere. So are pink (and lavender and blue and green) blankets of love.

Our main task is to remember to choose.

Questions for Reflection:

1. Consider any concerns you have about your physical well-being. List your fears or worries about that condition.

2. Do you have all the information you need? Have you been fully diagnosed by a health practitioner you trust? If not, think of this as an information-gathering phase. Put your fears on hold.

3. Now, call three (or more) friends or family members who love you. Ask them to wrap you in a blanket of love and protection as you gather information, undergo any medical tests or procedures you might need, or seek treatment from a holistic healer.

4. Find a good guided meditation tape and devote a half-hour each day to listening, relaxing, and envisioning yourself as whole and protected.

# Chapter 11: Showing Up

A friend once said of her grandmother, "She fully occupied the space where she stood." I was very young then, but I still thrill a little when I remember those words. I would have liked to have known that grandmother.

I've asked my clients a lot of questions through the years, but the question behind the question is always, "Are you fully occupying the space where you stand?"

In our youth, we spend a lot of time being invisible. We hide behind roles and rules and relationships. We sequester ourselves in pre-set agendas that satisfy family expectations, societal norms, and religious formulas. At midlife, we begin to get cranky with it all. We long to show up—to fully inhabit our lives.

What does it mean to fully show up? It means to make peace with the reality that the institutions and the organizations and the authority figures in whom we have placed our trust are just as flawed as we are. It means to know that our inner experience is just as valid as anyone else's. It means to step into our own authority.

We see people every day who aren't fully present. They seem to belong to another time, wearing the demeanor of some out-dated version of who they once were, or who they once wanted to be. They appear in the mall as aging women dressed as teenagers, or middle-aged men at the beach in bikini bathing suits. Or maybe the signals are more subtle than dress. You look into their faces and you sense an emptiness or a mask-like quality, as though they have been frozen in time.

Middle-aged people who are fully alive are a true delight to behold. Like my friend's grandmother, they fully occupy their space. They possess what someone has called "density"—- a sense of substance and soulfulness that invites others to be fully present. It is a presence that is good-humored yet unapologetic about the imprints of aging: Laugh-lines and spider veins and gray hair, while humbling, are the signs of well-earned wisdom, the fruits of a well-lived life.

I can remember the first time a sales clerk called me "ma'am" with that vacant-eyed look that is reserved for older people. I felt dismissed, unseen, and irritated. For awhile, I lamented living in a culture that worships youth and beauty—and then I began to re-think the problem. The truth was that I had not been fully present that day. Showing up is a primary task of life—and if you haven't done it by middle age, the task is no longer optional.

So how do we begin to fully show up?

We shift being a victim of circumstances to that of a full partner in a world we are helping to co-create. We begin to think of our experiences more in terms of what we've learned and how we've been blessed than in terms of what we've been through and how we've suffered.

We fully inhabit our bodies. We do it through a consciousness of a well-centered posture, of being aware that our body language communicates far more than words about who we are and what wisdom we hold. We cherish our bodies, knowing that they are the precious and finite vessels for our journey here on earth. We feed ourselves with good nutrients and strengthen ourselves with good exercise. We walk or we bicycle or we practice yoga or we dance—and we appreciate the sense of joyfulness that can come only from physical movement.

We remember that sometimes the best way to show up is to retreat for awhile. We honor our introverted selves—our need to dream, to sleep, to write, to be silent—in order to replenish our energy and listen more deeply.

We people our lives with friends and family members who are healthy, supportive, positive, and loving, and we commit ourselves to their growth as well as to our own.

We speak out clearly with well-measured words, but we listen more than we talk. We know that the deepest truths are sometimes best told in whispers, and that the most meaningful communication often happens in the pauses within conversation.

Sometimes the crises and losses of midlife force us to show up. A parent is diagnosed with Alzheimer's Disease. A spouse is disabled, or an adult child is struck with a mental illness. When trauma hits, we often revert to our victim stance: "This is too much. Why me? Who can I turn to? Who's the grown-up here?" And, after a (hopefully) brief regression into helplessness and despair, we realize that we are our own best authority. We allow ourselves time to grieve—but we also begin to educate ourselves about the challenges we face. We hire a coach or a therapist or a health care professional to companion us through the transition.

I don't know about you, but sometimes I get tired of being a grownup. On days when I feel depleted and saturated with the problems of midlife, I remember to call a caring friend. I schedule a "spirit day" for rest, for a long walk, for reading poetry, or for seeing a good movie. I buy myself some flowers and put them on my nightstand.

Lately I've been beleaguered with the demands of care-giving. A friend reminded me this week, "You don't need to work so hard at this. Skip the meeting, stay in bed, eat chocolate-chip cookies, make love with your husband." I was grateful for that nurturing voice.

Showing up, most of all, means finding balance. Pleasure and work. Giving and receiving. Introversion and extraversion. Showing up means knowing that self-respect and respect for others are not separate at all. They are equal and complementary parts of the great Round of Life of which we are a vital part.

Showing up means stepping into that Round with consciousness, dignity, and joy.

Questions for Reflection:

1. Which are the places in your past where you have felt the most vital and alive? Make note of them in your journal.

2. Now, think about your present life. Are there any situations that leave you feeling powerless or invisible?

3. What connection can you make between the two? What ingredients are needed right now to strengthen and empower you in the

*Daphne Stevens*

challenges you face? More time with your friends, a silent retreat, some additions to your wardrobe? Be as generous and detailed as you can.

# Chapter 12: Staying Awake

It may come in the moment when we learn of a friend's sudden demise of a heart attack while jogging. It may come when a parent with dementia fails to recognize us. Or it may come in the moment we discover the dreaded lump in our breast. In our middle years, death begins to present itself as a reality.

It may also come in small ways. We awaken on our fortieth birthday to realize that despite a lifetime devoted to health and fitness, we are peering into the mirror at a middle-aged face, and we are as close to sixty as we are to twenty. We try to get up on water-skis one summer, and we realize we don't have the strength we used to. Or the lady in the check-out line asks artlessly, "Do you get the senior-citizen discount?" Such moments are humbling, but they wake us up.

Sometimes mortality comes as a friend. We get weary of living in a world fraught with conflict and cruelty. The unrelenting realities of taxes and root canals and unsolvable family problems weigh us down. We consider the day when we will relinquish our burdens and cross over to another reality—and we discover that vision, not as a sign of despair or depression, but as anticipation of yet another life transition.

My own consciousness of death comes in stages. In my early twenties, I asked a wise friend and mentor what I needed to do to become a good therapist. He replied, "You need to learn to listen with all your pores open, to be fully present in the moment with all that you are. And you need to sit with the reality of your own death until it becomes your friend."

By my late thirties, my wise friend was dead. He had fought a long battle with lymphoma, but at 44, he was too young to die. I remember awakening each morning as if to a nightmare: How could it be that Jim was not in the world? Yet his presence has continued as companion and guide as I listen to the stories of my clients.

National tragedy reminds us of the presence of death in a particularly graphic way. In the aftermath of September 11, we watched again and again the replay of unspeakable devastation. A local news reporter asked me, "Why do we keep watching these images over and over?" I was feeling fatigued and impatient enough at the time to want to snap, "Because you people keep PLAYING them over and over!" But, instead, I deepened into the question.

We watch TV images of devastation, of course, partly because in our souls we want to make a connection between our inner realities and the outer world. We cannot take in the horrors of death and the pervasiveness of human atrocity, so we re-live them through the nightly news—but I believe that our fascination is more than grisly curiosity.

Our egos constantly say a loud NO to the reality that we are all here for a wink and then gone—but the truth is that our mortality is the only thing that keeps us awake and alive. In the weeks and months after a national tragedy, I notice a particular atmosphere of tenderness, even among strangers. People are more patient with one another in traffic. Neighbors who otherwise hardly speak to each other greet one another as kin. At such times we live in fear and shock— but we're also quickened to the preciousness of life, and the reality that, although we spend our lives scheming and dreaming and planning for our futures, the present is all we really have.

Late last fall, I was reminded of death in a very personal way when my husband and I were in a near-fatal car accident. The impact was quick and terrible, and as I sat, stunned, with bits and pieces of the shattered windshield in my lap and the acrid smell of deployed air bags in my nostrils, I thought absently, So this is how it ends. It's just this ordinary. One moment you're laughing, immersed in life, and sure of where you're going. The next moment you're sitting in the wreckage that used to be your car.

An awareness of my husband jerked me out of my stupor. He wasn't moving. My hands seemed to find his before I could will my eyes to register. I grabbed him, as if to force him back into consciousness. "Don't you dare leave me here," I whispered, stupid and fierce. After a wild ambulance ride and a lot of hours in an emergency room, we were both pronounced alive and well. We held each other tightly that night. Consciousness of his precious breathing permeated my dreams. I awoke at intervals, startling again and again at the memory of the impact of the wreck—and then relaxing into a rush of relief as I realized we were still on this earth together.

Ever since that day, I look into my husband's face with a renewed consciousness of the brevity of our stay here on earth, and of how blessed I am to be sharing my sojourn with him. This awakening to the divine ordinary is the gift that the presence of death gives us every day of our lives.

My mother has been diagnosed with Alzheimer's Disease, and I'm struggling. How can I be a good daughter now, knowing that the continuity of day- to-day conversations will no longer be the connecting thread between us? How can I offer comfort in a family where intellectual prowess and the illusion of control have been primary values? I respond to my parents in simple ways—the daily phone conversation, the drop-in visit, the endless consults with doctors and caregivers and other family members, as we try to sort out fear from reality and to plan the best course of care. But I respond, too, with a special kind of awareness. As I go for my daily walks, I take in the sweet smells of spring, the caress of the breeze, the green-ness of the sacred day with a special kind of wonder. I do it in honor of my mother's life—of all that is conscious and unconscious in her, of all that is lived and unlived about her essential being. I think of it as intercessory walking—of being conscious on her behalf—but it also serves something profound in me. I want to so permeate my body and my psyche with pleasure that when I die, the very cells of my cremated ashes in the earth will infuse the planet in some small way with the capacity for more aliveness.

Staying awake is both a gift and a task—the legacy of a life lived with death as a companion and teacher. We lose that legacy when we fall into a sentimentalized version of life that views death as wrong or personal or unjust or unfair. Midlife teaches us to be tender toward the parts of ourselves that are fearful or angry or even numb about death. It also teaches us to be shaped, molded, and deepened by its presence.

Questions for Reflection:

1. How do you experience the presence of death—as an inevitable process? a cruel intrusion? a numbing reality? Consider your own experiences with death, either in brushes with your own mortality, in the death of someone that you loved, or in the other personal losses you've suffered.

2. In your meditation or prayer practice, invite the presence of Death into your consciousness. How does it appear? See if you can have a conversation with this presence, and record it in your journal.

3. If this exercise is too jarring, skip it for now, or seek the help of a spiritual guide—a pastor or a spiritual director or a trusted friend. In the meantime, just entertain the possibility that death is a presence in your life that will continually remind you to stay awake to the preciousness of each moment here on earth.

# Chapter 13: Telling the Truth

There's a wonderful line from a terrible film called "The Russia House." Michelle Pfeiffer turns to Sean Connery and says in a fake Russian accent, "In my life now, I only have room for the truth." That one line was worth the cost of the video rental to me.

Truth-telling is a misunderstood and undervalued art. When I was young, I went around telling the truth indiscriminately. I idealistically and artlessly called attention to whatever inconsistencies and injustices offended my sensibilities. I jousted at windmills without regard for context. I was convinced that my well-meaning ego wisdom could serve to change institutions, enlighten clients, and motivate students. It is a magical thing to be bound and determined to change the world, and I remember that era with a delicious combination of nostalgia and chagrin.

As I grow older, I realize that, despite my best intentions, I have lived out many of the mistakes for which I criticized my parents. I've come to appreciate the eternity required to create a human being. I know that, in the context of that eternity, a year goes by in the blink of an eye. A sense of timelessness prevails for me. I know that planning and living into visions are, in reality, hand-work to keep myself busy so that my soul can get on with the work of unfolding. The ancient alchemists experimented endlessly trying to turn base metal into gold, and through the process of that seemingly futile work, their consciousness was transformed. As a modern alchemist, I plan out my life in the effort to turn the base metal of possibility into the gold of realized dreams. As I step through the paces toward a more fulfilled life, I come to know that the real work is not the achievement of my ego's best plans—it is the work of my own transformation.

Transformation, of course, never happens in a vacuum. We need friends who appreciate the subtleties of our unfolding souls—friends who tell the truth when truth serves the emergence of our higher selves.

The Buddhists have a name for this kind of companionship: a Noble Friend. A Noble Friend is one who looks into your eyes and sees you at your neediest, your pettiest, your finest, and your wisest, and doesn't see a discrepancy among all of those selves. A Noble Friend is one who dares to risk the loss of your friendship when she senses you need to hear a truth, because she knows that both you and she belong to something much greater than yourselves. A Noble Friend can celebrate your highest achievements without envy. She knows that you and she are a part of a great mosaic of humanity, and that, when light shines through your particular gifts, her gifts are illuminated as well.

My friend Barbara is a Noble Friend. We have companioned each other for thirty years now, celebrating weddings, grieving the deaths of mutual friends, encouraging one another through pregnancies, and rejoicing at births and graduations. We have traveled long distances to attend milestone birthday parties and the christenings of grandchildren. We have laughed, marveled occasionally at the brilliance of our own conversation, and both lamented and welcomed the inevitable ways that our shadow-selves periodically show up to confuse and enlighten us. I'm not sure why Barbara has hung around with me for three decades, but I know why I cherish her kinship. Barbara is a truth-teller.

I remember a moment when I was in the worst depression of my life. My marriage of some seventeen years had just dissolved. I had a stack of bills and a leaking roof, my daughter was ill, and I was feeling pretty hopeless. Barbara and I were in daily contact by phone, doing the things that women do in the face of grief. We wept. We reminisced. We talked about our dreams. We compared notes on how to rebuild our lives, and how to raise teenagers alone. There were countless tender moments between us in that long season of sadness—but I remember one in particular.

I was agonizing over some detail or other, getting caught up in the drama of my own suffering. Barbara's voice was crisp. "Well," she said gently. "Don't get too attached to your misery."

My first response was to feel insulted. How dare she minimize my struggle? But even in that moment, I realized how profoundly she respected me. She didn't accept the idea that I was too weak or pitiful to meet the challenges that life was piling onto my plate. She was willing to listen to endless complaints, but she wasn't willing to let me succumb to victim-hood. I felt a little like a character in an old melodrama who, slapped in the face, is released from hysteria. "Thanks, I needed that," became a mantra. "Thanks, I needed that" became a reminder that I was truly more than the sum of my troubles. It was a gift that only a Noble Friend could deliver.

*Watercolor Bedroom*

Telling the truth is always a gift, but there are some secrets about it that young people don't know. Truth-telling is a privilege, not a right. It is earned through long decades of building friendships. It is earned through a lifetime of learning painstakingly that the best truths are often told through silence, and that a few well-placed words are more powerful than a passionate sermon. It is earned through a life of communing with nature, of reading the great poets, of listening and discerning the truths embedded in the words of others—and through listening to the symbolic language of imagination and dreams.

"In my life now, I only have room for the truth." Some days that's true for me, and sometimes I still get attached to the drama of suffering for its own sake. But, with the help of my community of Noble Friends, I am learning to so immerse myself in the pleasures of ordinary days that the lies that trigger anxiety and worry just don't have room to take root.

Questions for Reflection:

1. Who are the truth-tellers in your life? Remember the moments when they have called you home to yourself and your strengths. If you're still in contact with them, consider writing a note or an email, thanking them for the role they have played in shaping the course of your life.

2. What do you know about your truth-telling abilities? Do you tend to gloss over difficulties? To stone-wall and then bombard your loved ones with complaints? Just as an experiment, spend the next week acknowledging truth and avoiding lies. You don't always have to tell the

*Daphne Stevens*

whole truth, of course—but remember that telling falsehoods will diminish your energy and weaken you.

# Chapter 14: Letting Go

There's an oft-repeated bit of shamanic wisdom that is told as a four-part lesson for living in peace with oneself and the world. It goes something like this: 1. Show up. 2. Stay awake. 3. Tell the truth. 4. Let go of the outcome.

I have to admit that I understand the first three better than I do the fourth. "Let go of the outcome." It flows off the tongue so easily, until we are faced with a real or imagined threat: An adult child creates a crisis. A client expresses dissatisfaction. A friend betrays a major confidence. How do we let go of outcome in those moments—when we feel wronged, unsafe, when we are filled with anger?

Forgiveness is one way. Forgiveness feels like an impossible task when we have been betrayed by someone we trust. But betrayals—both the big hurts that change our lives and the little hurts that sully our days—are crucial to both growth and change. Betrayals force us to let go of dependencies that no longer serve us. The intuitive healer Caroline Myss has suggested that betrayals "shake our faith in human justice and the social code and move us to place our trust in the chaotic justice of the Divine." This shift is crucial in midlife, when we must move beyond a child's insistence that faith is related to fairness in order to move into our rightful role as an elder in the tribe.

Most people say, "I can't imagine forgiving him/her" when what they mean is "I can't imagine forgetting this." But forgiving doesn't require forgetting. Forgetting is silly when we have the opportunity to learn a great lesson—and it is usually impossible when we have been hurt. My friend Cindy, a Native American medicine woman, suggests a unique response that speaks to the wisdom of remembering. "Thank you for revealing yourself to me," she is known to say in the face of a betrayal. "Now I will know how to take care of myself better."

But forgiving goes beyond not-forgetting. It requires nothing more (or less) than relinquishing our assumption that we know everything about another person's inner world. It requires giving up the delusion that we know all about the motivations, struggles, and ambiguities that have influenced the situation that has wounded us. It requires opening ourselves to the possibility that we are part of a story that is about something larger than our own ideas about rightness and wrongness.

"It's all about me." I saw the sentence on a T-shirt in a local boutique. I noticed a couple of things about that shirt. It was stocked in baby blue, hanging next to a bunch of pink ones that that said "Princess." And it only came in pre-teen sizes.

Forgiveness obliges us to turn loose of our "It's all about me" T-shirt. It invites us to move from inner conversations about Justice (Was this fair? Was I right or wrong? Am I 'crazy,' or is he/she?) and move into inner conversations about Love. Turning the other cheek is not some namby-pamby action designed to invite further betrayal. Turning the other cheek simply means doing something interesting instead of doing something predictable.

"'Vengeance is mine' saith the Lord." It's often used as a proof-text describing God as a punitive angry father-figure who is more interested in justice than love. I'm not a theologian, but as I get older, I wonder if another way to look at that text is this: Vengeance is predictable. It's burdensome. It's boring. God is willing to carry the burden of justice so that we poor beleaguered human beings don't have to. Because God is carrying the burden of balancing the scales in whatever way they need to be balanced, we can be free to be generous with ourselves and one another. We can do something interesting. We can turn the other cheek or kiss each other on the head. We can say, in Cindy's words, "Thank you for revealing yourself to me." And maybe—just maybe—we can let go of the burden of being right and accept the gift of being happy instead.

Forgiveness—letting go— is a radical action. It cuts to the quick of our most fervent beliefs about ourselves: Can it be that my worth, value, or safety is truly not in the hands of another person? Do I dare to let go of the idea that, unless the other person "gets the point" and suffers the way he or she has made me suffer, I will not be secure? Or, more to the point, is it possible that I can be okay and not be in control of another person's behavior?

Letting go. Forgiving. It's a task, it's a gift, and it's a luxury.

Questions for Reflection:
1. Think about someone who has recently hurt you in some way.
2. Consider what you want to do in response— "set them straight," have the last word, pay them back, or write them off.

3. Now, instead of doing something predictable like that, ask "What would be a more interesting response?"

4. Make a response that has absolutely nothing to do with expectations or control of their behavior. Your purpose here is to set yourself free and to expand your repertoire of responses to life's challenges.

5. Celebrate your freedom with a concrete action, and look for other possibilities for building graciousness and spontaneity into your life.

# Chapter 15: Easter Morning

I'm probably going to blow my cover here, but I am not a sentimentalist. I sneer at syrupy greeting cards. I scoff at sappy love songs. To me, sentimentalism as an anemic version of passion—and anemia is not very life-giving.

Teresa, a special friend of mine in graduate school, appreciated my misanthropic bent. "You're the only person I know," she once said, "with whom I can meet for an hour over a beer and evoke the spirit of Ash Wednesday, Maundy Thursday, and Good Friday and all of the other dark holidays. You understand holy paradox as well as anyone I know."

I was honored. Holy paradox is something I treasure. It can't be shared with just anyone. I mean, how can I profess to know without a doubt the existence of a loving God, and at the same time hold everything in reserve about what He (She?) is purported to have ever said? How can I stay in a continual state of wonder at God's creation, and simultaneously growl at the blindness and short-sightedness of my fellow human beings? And, while I'm at it, how can I basically feel as humble as I do, and at the same time write boldly about these things?

But I have a confession to make, to Teresa and the other cronies with whom I periodically share a sacramental beer and evoke the spirit of the Dark Holy Days. I am crazy about Easter.

I love Easter because it is one of the few holidays in the Christian calendar that hasn't been totally distorted by consumerism. I give Norman

Rockwell personal credit for this. I mean, the man imprinted us with images of what the perfect Christmas should look like. We are collectively burdened by the pictures of beatific families gathered around holiday tables—the wise faces of the elders, the ecstasy of the little ones who can't wait to get past the family meal and into the festivities to come. Old Norman even set the menu for us. I mean, you haven't experienced a proper Christmas in this country unless you have eaten turkey, replete with dressing and cranberry jelly, pumpkin pie, and "all the fixings," as they say.

I object to such formulaic images. When I line up, sheep-like, at the local grocery, to purchase the obligatory turkey in December, I feel vaguely confused, as if I'm a character in somebody else's play. Or I buck the system, preparing an elaborate Chinese dinner on Christmas Eve, only to endure baleful looks from my now-grown kids. No turkey? Mom must be having hot flashes again. Christmas, after all, isn't Christmas without Christmas food.

Which leads me to what I love about Easter. Easter is a high holy day, like Christmas. But, unlike Christmas, Easter isn't pre-orchestrated by the powers that be who decide what makes for a suitable holiday. I mean, nobody says, "Have you gotten your Easter shopping done yet?" weeks before the appointed date. And nobody bemoans the fact on Good Friday that they haven't finished their Easter decorating. Nobody bores their friends and relatives with an elaborate Easter newsletter. What warmed-over news could compete with the message inherent in the real Easter story?

Easter, at its most secular, says, "Hooray! The long winter has melted into glorious spring. The colors are splendid. The sun and the rain bless the flowers and the crops so no one can miss the miracle of the season." And Easter, at its most religious, says, "Hallelujah! Our God is a God who has risen from the dead. He brings the spring-time with His glorious Resurrection."

Easter, in my mind, invites a more personal response than any other holiday. For one thing, a festival that hasn't been hopelessly distorted by the culture allows us to be creative. What is your favorite way to celebrate spring? In a church scented with incense and resounding with choral music? In the woods by a stream on the first camping trip of the season? In your garden, smelling the moist sweet earth and witnessing the first tentative splash of color from the bulbs you planted last fall?

The Easter story itself elicits something unique and personal. I can easily embrace the notion of a Divine Child being born on a cold winter's night. I've known cold winters, and I've held newborns in my arms. I've even fancied that I heard the sound of angel choirs in the cooing and laughter of tiny cherubs in my life.

But Easter? A dead man, scarred with holes through his hands and feet, just walks right out of his own tomb. He is fully himself, yet he is unrecognizable to his closest friends. "Fear not," he says—he always says that. But those same friends scatter in terror. How can we not fear when the dead are suddenly alive among us?

The story of Easter challenges us to let go of our white-knuckled notions about what is real. We might be able to gloss over the notion of the

Virgin Birth—it's only mentioned in two of the four Gospel accounts, and we can tell ourselves that it doesn't matter anyway. But the Resurrection is a bedrock of our faith tradition. In its story, God, the great Rule-Maker who created order out of the chaos, declares, "The Rules don't matter! They don't bring you life! What brings you life is not the preconceived beliefs that you hold. What brings you life is your infinite, God-given capacity to be surprised!" Easter, then, is the ultimate surprise, celebrated anew with each coming spring.

My friend Dan Edwards has expressed it well. "The point is not that Jesus walked out of his tomb," he says. "That really doesn't matter—unless you *yourself* walk out of your own personal tomb."

What are the places in your life where you are stuck—entombed by old beliefs about yourself? Where are the places you are trapped in lifeless relationship patterns, or even in a religion so deadly serious that it holds no promise for surprise, for humor, or for playfulness? Each year, Father Dan poses that question in a subtly different play of words. And each year I realize some perception that I have elevated into my version of ultimate truth, closing myself to the possibility of a mystery that is ever-unfolding—a mystery as intricate and delicate and colorful as the irises that bloom outside my bedroom window on this Easter morning.

Questions for Reflection:

1. In what ways do you celebrate spring? Brainstorm in your journal all the ways you have invited the season into your life. (Spring

cleaning, outdoor activities, a trip to the beach, planting a garden are just a few.)

2. How does your religious tradition serve you in saying yes to the season? If you're a Christian, how does Easter express itself best to you? If you're of another tradition, how do the rituals and stories of your faith help you to celebrate spring?

3. How does your self-care reflect the changing of the season? Buying a new spring wardrobe? Rearranging your closet? Treating yourself to a skin peel to slough off the dead skin of winter? Polishing your toenails in preparation for sandal-weather?

4. What worn-out beliefs or practices are you letting go of this season? In what ways have you been surprised, by your own gifts or by the gifts of others in your life, or by synchronistic events that allow you to feel more fully alive this spring?

5. Jot these things down in your journal. Take action to fully enjoy the change of the seasons.

## Chapter 16: Unfinished Children

"If only I could get my daughter to a healthier place," a mother recently commented, "then I could get on with my life." Her devotion is admirable, but her logic is faulty. She is dealing with an adult Unfinished Child.

When you are traveling with a toddler on an airplane, the first rule of safety is this: In the event of a loss of cabin pressure, put on your own oxygen mask before you put on your child's. The rule is the same when dealing with Unfinished Children. When we bypass our own needs, rescuing and fixing, we needlessly sacrifice ourselves and we don't help our children. How can we remember to put on our own oxygen masks before we try to help those we love?

For some fortunate people, the launching phase of child-rearing is a time of adjustment and re-focusing. But for parents with Unfinished Children—young adults who are afflicted with mental illness, addiction, learning problems, or chronic immaturity—the question of who gets the oxygen mask first can be a matter of survival for both generations.

Right responses, of course, are different for every family, but hard experience taught me some principles for parenting young adults:

**1. Foster responsibility.** It's crucial to hold our adult children accountable for whatever they can do for themselves. Accountability may mean calling the law when an Unfinished Child threatens to abuse people or property. It may mean house rules that require the homebound to get outside at least once a day or take medicines on time or attend a support group. It may require that any financial support be contingent on an adult child staying in school. Your values and your comfort level will determine what accountability means in your particular household.

**2. Be realistic about limitations.** As much as I love my adult children, it wasn't feasible past a certain point for them to live in my house. At times, I even needed to limit my contact with them.

**3. Know that guilt and self-deprivation never launched an Unfinished Child.** I had to make sure to get ample sleep, exercise, and good nutrition. I nurtured relationships with my husband and friends. I wanted to be a good example for my children by seeking health and wholeness in every way I could.

**4. Seek spiritual help.** I sensed that unsolvable problems would either deepen my relationship with God or mire me into despair and self-pity. Personal prayer, spiritual direction, the sacramental space of a church community, and 12-Step groups provided much-needed comfort and support.

**5. Fill your life with as much beauty, play, and creativity as you can find.** Some days this was an enormous task for me, but dealing with troubled adult children drains energy. I began to go spiritually and emotionally bankrupt whenever I failed to replenish my own inner resources, so I learned to attend to myself more deeply.

**6. Seek psychotherapy and coaching to help navigate through the challenges.** With help, I clarified my own goals and developed a plan for envisioning a life beyond the painful present.

**7. Talk to your spouse.** By agreeing on boundaries for the children, my husband and I were gradually freed from the crippling cycle of guilt, anger, frustration and exhaustion.

Unfinished Children were the challenge of my life. Those hard years forced me to move beyond shame, outrage, and self-pity into a deeper kind of knowing and a larger kind of love. Through the years of letting go of old scripts and embracing new realities, I was able to bless my children and accept the unfinished places within myself. I learned to respect my children and the paths they have chosen— the lives that they are creating for themselves.

Questions for Reflection:

1. If you are the parent of an Unfinished Child, use your journal to express your feelings of frustration, anxiety, guilt, and rage. Know that your feelings are completely normal. Negative feelings don't mean you don't love your child, and they are likely to change as time goes by.

2. Notice your feelings as indications of your human limitations— nothing more.

3. In *For Mothers of Difficult Daughters,* Charney Hurst observes that our culture—including mental health professionals—can be brutal in its assumption that mothers of Unfinished Children are more flawed than other people, to be blamed somehow for their children's problems. If you seek therapy, avoid clinicians with such a bias.

*Watercolor Bedroom*

4. Draw upon relationships with people you trust—your partner or your pastor or friends, especially other women who have struggled (and hopefully resolved issues) with Unfinished Children.

5. Try to limit your contact with your adult children to times when you feel rested and collected. Remember that your spiritual and emotional health will provide solid role models and hope for them, even when they are showing you nothing but defiance.

6. If you are blessed with healthy adult children, be supportive of friends who may be struggling. When I was in the worst part of my pain, I received a simple card from a woman I knew from a yoga class. It read, "If life were a school, you'd deserve a recess!" I'll always be grateful for the kindness of that woman.

*Daphne Stevens*

# Chapter 17: Radical Self-Care

Sometimes I get irritated with everybody I know. Nothing I do is quite right, and I drive myself harder and harder to make up for things I can't fix. One of the benefits of getting older is having the sense to give up the struggle a lot sooner than I used to.

I hear women say self-disparaging things like "I'm PMS-ing" to describe such times, and then I feel even more annoyed: When did "PMS-ing" become a verb? Why is it that we discredit the signals of our bodies and our souls—those symptoms that tell us we have abandoned ourselves and fallen prey to the temptation to live someone else's life instead of our own? When did we start diagnosing ourselves instead of listening to our inner wisdom?

Young motherhood taught me a great deal about listening. Like all children, my daughter could be subject to exhaustion and bad temper, and I learned that some things weren't helpful. Being judgmental was the worst response I could give. Reacting out of my own frustration only compounded the problem. I found that covering certain basics was the only sane response. Was she hungry? Was she too hot or cold? Did she need a nap or a warm soothing bath or some time reading stories in our big recliner? Did she need a time-out to calm down and rest? The checklist seems too obvious to miss, but it always took an intentional focus to remember those basics before moving further.

When we get tired, we're like cranky toddlers, but most of us aren't very kind to ourselves. When I ask women about self-care, they often get apologetic. "I don't exercise like I should," they confess. Or, even more self-disparaging, "I eat like a pig." Or, with a tone of subtle self-justification, "Sleep? Who has time to sleep? I get six hours if I'm lucky." I tell my clients, "If you were to discount your children's needs the way you do your own, I'd have to call Protective Services. If you were as mean to them as you are to yourself, I'd call it neglect or abuse."

"Stress management" was one of the many buzz-words of the 80s and 90s. On the surface, it seemed like an answer. After all, we *were* over-stressed. We believed that, if we stayed focused on stringent programs of physical fitness and relaxation training and creative visualization and the "self-nurturing" dates we penciled into our overcrowded appointment books, we could somehow do it all. We could balance childcare and family obligations and community activities and careers. We could break through the "glass ceiling" and take the "mommy track" to high levels of achievement.

We believed that we could keep our sanity if we devoured enough self-help books about how (or how not) to be superwomen.

I totally bought the myth. When I got overwhelmed and fatigued and cranky, I attributed it to my own inadequacy. "PMS" wasn't a verb back then, but it sure was a syndrome—and while it was helpful to know about my own cycles of mood and energy, PMS became one more way of diagnosing myself in order to avoid the reality that it was all just *too much*. Self-care was a euphemism for throwing myself a bone—just enough rest or nutrition or exercise to drive myself like a pack animal into the next bout of frenzied activity. Life was about doing—accomplishing and achieving—and the list was ever-growing.

Midlife women know a lot about this dilemma, and we need to share what we know. I can't take away the overwork of my young mother friends, but I can gently remind them that they are doing the impossible. I can suggest that, at best, this is a time for making more conscious choices—and that, at worst, this time will pass. If I am careful about my own energy and efforts, I can even help them out on occasion. I can provide child-care for the church nursery. Or I can spend an hour or an afternoon with a tiny friend or grandchild to give a beleaguered mother some much-needed relief.

But we can't be nurturing wise-women until we've fully stepped into our authority. We have to live our lives from the center of our own beings before we can be of service to others. We have to practice what I call radical self-care.

What is radical self-care? It is a discipline we each discover for ourselves, and there are no hard and fast rules. Radical self-care is present in the acts of kindness we offer ourselves the way we'd offer a child an ice cream cone in summer or an extra blanket on a chilly night. It has to do with the things we do just for the delight of doing them. I practice radical self-care whenever I take a walk on a crisp fall morning or a nap on a rainy afternoon. I practice it when I read a book just for pleasure, when I luxuriate on a massage table, or when I savor the taste of a truly good meal. I practice it psychically when I take time in the mornings to write down my dreams before starting my day, and I practice it spiritually when I resist the temptation to be self-apologetic or to justify myself to others.

Radical self care is a courageous practice. It means resisting the illusion that we can earn our space on the planet by sacrificing ourselves. It means letting go of "PMS-ing" in order to drop into self-indulgence and stay there until we are enfolded with a sense of grace—of being loved, not because we've earned it through our suffering but just because we are.

Questions for Reflection:

1. When was the last time you felt truly rested and cared-for, fit and well-fed and content?

2. If it's been more than a week, move into a radical self-care mode. If you need to clear your calendar to make room for yourself, do so as early as possible. Take naps, walk in the woods, go to a museum, have a massage—any act of self-love that you might do for a child or a good friend who is exhausted.

3. Write a dialogue in your journal between your well-cared-for self and your loving Mother self. See if those different voices have something to say to each other about continuing the practice of radical self-care.

*Daphne Stevens*

# Chapter 18: Holy Commerce

I shopped like a madwoman last month. Why is it easier to fit new clothes into a suitcase than to drag out the season's old favorites and wear them again? I was preparing for a business trip to Santa Fe. First I hit some tried-and-true catalogs for basics—good fitting pants in several neutral colors, and a simple packable dress that could be accessorized easily. Then I hit the mall.

I don't do the mall very often. It overwhelms me. By the time I bought tunics to go with my catalogue pants and then searched the outlet stores to find shells to go under the tunics, I was pretty exhausted.

I have a recurring dream about being in a shop surrounded by beauty— exquisite fabrics and jewelry in an infinite assortment of colors and textures. In Santa Fe I lived that dream. Santa Fe is famous for its shopping, but what I enjoyed the most was a long walkway where Native American artisans display their goods. They sit on the ground with the work of their hands arranged on blankets in front of them. I was captivated by the vibrant display, but I was equally enchanted by the faces of the artists themselves.

I felt shy. I am accustomed to American mall shopping. You know, you breeze in and sort through rack after rack of the same name-brand style you've seen in the last store and the one before that. You might have even found something close to what you like three stores back, but you're

*Watercolor Bedroom*

looking for a better price or a different color, or you can't find the pants that went with the jacket you found earlier.

The displays are basically the same. The same bored-looking sales clerk stares at you. She may be old and tired or she may be young and impatient, but she is seldom helpful. "Just make up your mind," her manner says. You finally pick out something close to what you were looking for and position yourself in the back of the check-out line. Or you ask, "Do you have any of these in a different size?" and the sales clerk switches from bored to annoyed. "Everything we have is out," she might say. You feel extraneous, invisible, as if you've asked too much. Maybe you get annoyed back. Or maybe you're so numbed by the day's rush of stimuli that you don't even notice the emptiness of the exchange.

I wasn't fully aware of the soul of shopping until I walked that walkway in Santa Fe and looked into the faces of the merchants there. They had created each piece they offered. There was a story behind each beaded necklace, a signature of style in each pottery selection.

I was looking for a turquoise choker for myself and a birthday gift for my good friend Beth. I was looking for the perfect pair of cuff-links for my husband. As I stopped and examined each choice, a gentle exchange transpired. No bored or impatient (or eager) salesperson met my eye—only a simple earth-dweller like me. A sense of dignity and a mutual respect prevailed as I gazed into each brown and weathered face.

It got me to thinking about buying and selling. Mass production and retail has given us a lot. I'm happy to have a car and a refrigerator—and, yes, I'm even happy to have access to those racks of clothes in the mall. But consumerism gives us illusion as much as it gives us choice. We grab armloads of clothes to try on, forgetting that some human being in some distant place actually worked with a piece of fabric to produce those dresses. We forget that a human being— a designer or some designer's assistant—had some idea that became manifest in this jacket. We forget, too, that the bored-looking sales clerk may also be a mother or a student or a poet or a prophet. That all the hands that worked to bring us this purchase are earth-dwellers— just like us.

My husband has a bit of wisdom about money. He says, "I think money has three purposes. It is there to empower us to take care of our basic needs. It is there to give us pleasure. And it is there to enable us to bring both to others—both basic needs and pleasure. That last thing, I think, is the best thing about any kind of wealth."

I couldn't agree with him more. Money embodies our very life substance—the time and energy that is given to us to spend here on earth. Greed is not money, after all, any more than gluttony is food. It's all good, as the kids say, in its own time and place.

I considered all that as I looked into the eyes of the young Santa Fe artist and offered my money in exchange for a beautiful turquoise necklace. There was reverence and a hint of joy in both the buying and in the selling.

I think that I will wear that necklace often.

*Watercolor Bedroom*

Questions for Reflection:

1. How often do you look into the face of a sales clerk when you are buying something? What do you see there?

2. Spend some time this week being conscious of exactly how you spend your money. How do you see those purchases as supportive of your basic human values? How many of those purchases provide for your basic needs—or give you pleasure—or afford pleasure or necessities for others?

3. What is your notion of tithing? How are you conscious of giving back to a community, a world, or a Divine Being from which you have drawn strength?

## Chapter 19: Mother's Day

"What are you doing for your mother for Mother's Day?" It was a question that got tossed among co-workers when we were in our twenties and thirties, inevitable as the coming of warm weather. It was a difficult question for most of us, except the few who enjoyed living in families who were warm and not too complicated. Those lucky few sailed blissfully through Mother's Day—or else they lied about it. The rest of us deliberated throughout April.

We were filled with clever ideas for thoughtful gestures and gifts. The problem was that most of us were so tentative about our fledgling status that we couldn't stand too much mother-connection. I mean, where was a card or gift that conveyed, "I love you, but I'm working through my Mother Issues now and I have some ambivalence about you, and also some lack of clarity about where you end and where I begin. I want to tell you that I love you, but I don't want you to misunderstand what Love means for me this year. I want to acknowledge you, but I also need to find my own path. I'm not sure you're willing to honor my right to find my own path, and that kind of pisses me off. I want you to know that I'm pissed off—but what I want you to know most of all is that my pissed-off-ness doesn't mean I don't love you."

I mean, does FDS offer a flower arrangement that conveys all of that?

I know a few young women who have made creative attempts that doubtlessly confused their poor mothers no end. One classic example is the young woman, caught in a pseudo-mutual and anxiously over-close maternal relationship, who sent a card that said, "You've been like a mother to me." Another young woman, in a more overtly toxic bond, sent her mom a Venus Fly Trap from the florist.

Ambivalence about our mothers has been around since the first teenage girl rolled her eyes and said, "*Mo-ther*," in that universal language of love commingled with disgust that is unique to mothers and daughters. Nancy Friday gave voice to the problem in the 1970s with a book called *My Mother Myself*. It sent millions of women to shrinks and to consciousness-raising groups with two questions that became mantras in that era: "How can I keep from being like *her*?" and "Why aren't she and I closer?"

One cure for that ambivalence is to raise our own daughters. Oh, the cure doesn't show up for the first eight years or so, while they are adorable and snuggly. But as we realize that our pre-pubescent daughters are looking at us with the same blend of disdain and embarrassment that characterized our feelings about our own mothers, we begin to re-consider things.

It's a pivotal point in a woman's life. If she chooses anger toward her daughter, she perpetuates a cycle of self-pity—the "Where did I go wrong?" syndrome that is far too common in middle aged women. If she chooses self-blame, she falls into an equally destructive trap, becoming a doormat for her daughter forever. Both pathways are equally death-producing—but, happily, there is a third way.

When a daughter begins the crucial and treacherous path toward individuation, we can recognize eye-rolling and defiance for what it is. We can say to ourselves, "Of *course* she'd rather fight with me than come face to face with the terrors of growing up and facing the world. And of *course* I feel abandoned and rejected." When we acknowledge both realities with a measure of equanimity, we bless ourselves and our daughters alike.

But how do we maintain our composure when the child of our heart rages against us with a vehemence that would become Attila the Hun?

We count to ten a lot. We remind ourselves, "Of course she's not grateful. How would she know to be grateful? Fish don't know they're in water. She can't know how much she's loved." We commiserate with our middle-aged friends. If we are especially lucky and our own mothers are available to us, we turn to them, and healing begins to happen.

My daughter, engaged to a wonderful man named Joe, is walking through a mine-field lately. Joe's daughter is fraught with unresolved feelings about her parents' divorce, and she is edging into puberty. It's a daunting challenge for any stepmother-to-be, and my daughter is stepping up to the plate. She called me recently with a litany of complaints. "I can't do anything right," she wailed. "She complains incessantly. She pouts. She plays me against her father. But you know what I hate most of all?"

"No," I murmured with genuine sympathy, "What do you hate most of all?"

"Mom. She rolls her *eyes* at me."

I suppressed a giggle and struggled to keep my voice neutral. "She rolls her eyes? Oh, I hate it when they do that."

"Yes, she rolls her eyes." Her voice became indignant. "I mean, no adult would have put up with that from me! How can she be so rude?"

I could no longer suppress the giggle. I said, "Honey. You rolled your eyes at me from the time you were seven until the time you were fifteen. You only stopped then because you learned to say, 'Screw you, Mom! I hate you!' Kate is precocious like you were, that's all."

We talked about the dangers of motherhood and the perils of step-motherhood. We laughed. We cried. We raged against the gods who give us children and make us love them unconditionally only to make them blind to the care we give them.

And I felt us both being enveloped by something larger—the presence, perhaps, of a Mother greater than the two of us, who has loved us enough to let us be ourselves and to learn to appreciate one another in moments like these.

Motherhood may be the ultimate opportunity for learning forgiveness of self and forgiveness of another. It is absolutely crucial to be able to say, all in one breath, "I failed you. I did my absolute best. I love you. You've hurt me. You're doing your best. We're both absolutely wonderful and terrible all at the same time."

It's as impossible and miraculous as birth.

Questions for reflection:

1. What are the ways you have felt abandoned by your mother? Where are the places you have felt affirmed and supported by her?

2. How do you see those patterns being re-played with your daughter, or your step-daughter, or your daughter-in law?

3. Write a letter in your journal to your un-mothered self—that part of you that feels orphaned, unseen or abused or abandoned. Reassure that Orphan within you that you will not allow her to be hurt any more.

4. Consider the relationships in which you feel child-like or helpless—a boss who is critical perhaps, or an acquaintance with whom you find yourself feeling diminished in some way. How can you protect yourself in those relationships by re-claiming your abandoned child and honoring your yearnings for belonging?

5. Write a note of appreciation to the women in your life with whom you have found healing—perhaps your mother or your daughter, or a woman friend who has mothered you in some way. Decide which notes to mail, and which to simply ponder in your heart as part of your own process of giving birth to yourself.

## Chapter 20: Dancing Lessons

One of the things I enjoy about my husband is his ability to surprise me. Last month I came home from work to find him poring over travel brochures. "How about a river boat cruise?"

I hesitated. "It's a Big Band cruise," he added. "We'd be dancing every night for a whole week."

Now, my idea of a vacation is NOT to be confined to a boat with a million other people and exorbitant amounts of rich food. I feel fat and claustrophobic at the very thought of it. But I do love good music—and I love to dance, even though I do it badly. "Great idea," I responded. "Very romantic. The only problem is that we're terrible dancers."

The next day held another surprise. "I've researched the Dance Question," my husband announced. "I've signed us up for three introductory lessons with a guy who swears he can teach us."

Now, my Dance History is a painful one. My mother dutifully carted me to Cotillion classes at age twelve—it was just what was *done* back in those days. I took from a lady called Miss Betty who showed us how to lumber through the basics of the Foxtrot and the Jitterbug, but whose main agenda, it seemed, was to socialize us to be Young Ladies and Young Gentlemen. Young Ladies were instructed to purr, "I'd *love* to," when asked to dance by Young Gentleman. A simple yes or no seemed plenty good enough for me, but I figured Miss Betty knew what she was talking about and I went along with the program. But then she repeatedly cued us Young Ladies to say, "You dance *divinely*." It would have seemed silly enough (I mean, who said *divinely*, even in the early 60s?)—but it was made utterly ridiculous by the fact that I was about two feet taller than most of the Young Gentlemen and I felt like the biggest lummox to ever (not) grace a dance floor. I mean, how could I look down at the Young Gentleman whose feet I was trouncing (and who invariably seemed to be staring straight at my breasts) and say "You dance *divinely*" with a straight face? It was the birth of feminist consciousness for me—but at least I learned a few steps.

I did pretty well during the late 60s and 70s. I mean, all we were doing was gyrating to Motown during the fast numbers and doing what I called the "shuffle and grope" during the slower, more romantic tunes. It didn't take a lot of skill to do either. But I always longed to really dance.

The next chapter came when my husband and I decided to venture onto the dance floor together shortly after we were married. The teacher this time was named Miss Polly. Now, Miss Polly was an excellent dancer, that was plain. I envied her every time she chose a partner from among the more accomplished members of the class and Tangoed or Jitterbugged or Waltzed her way through an ethereal cloud that transformed the YMCA gym into the set of a Fred Astaire movie. But the truth is that Miss Polly was a terrible teacher.

Miss Polly's primary teaching methods were demonstration and shame. If you didn't get the demonstration enough to ease into the progression of steps, she immediately made an example of you. My husband and I are practically the poster children for middle aged dyslexia:

We were *wonderful* examples for Miss Polly. "Aaron! Daphne!" Miss Polly would exclaim, exasperated, as we galloped around the floor in some grotesque imitation of what we thought we had seen her show us. *"He's supposed to be leading! Let's try that again—"* at which point we'd be the focal point of another Demonstration during which my poor husband would be dragged, sweating and panting, around the floor, trying to keep up with Miss Polly. Later, Miss Polly abandoned all pretense of trying to do remedial work; her reprimands were abbreviated to something like: "Don't do it the way Aaron and Daphne are doing it!" (She said my husband's name like "*AAAH*-ron," in a voice that sounded vaguely like a buzz saw cutting through slate.) Each scolding accelerated our mutual startle-reflex and intensified the unpleasantness of the whole ordeal.

It didn't take us long to decide we didn't want to stay under Miss Polly's tutelage. Fortunately, mid-lifers can laugh about experiences that would be devastating to younger, more tender egos. We decided that, although our intentions were good, dancing just might not be our gift.

Now, given this traumatic history, you can understand what a big deal it was when my husband announced that he was ready to give dancing another shot.

We arrived at our first lesson with a man named Mister Duncan. (Why is it that dancing teachers never have real names?) The lesson was designed to take us through a simple step, first without music, then with music, and then circulating throughout the room, trying it with other students. Mister Duncan apparently knows something about learning theory. He emphasizes very small steps, repetition, and frequent shifts from one mode to another in such a way that his students don't get bored. Most of all, he keeps the anxiety level low. "Don't worry about remembering any of this," he says. "It's your job to forget everything you learn when you leave here. It's my job to remind you." And, "It takes doing something five hundred times to make a muscle memory." I figure we're at about 67 repetitions each for every step we're learning—and the amazing fact is that, even at this stage, we're beginning to enjoy dancing together.

So all of this brings me to a few basic points. I love being at a point in life when I can learn new things without having to excel at anything. I also love being at a place where I can be wise about whom I entrust to teach me any given skill. And I love being free to simply enjoy movement and rhythm and music for its own sake—just because it's fun to move and play.

I also love being surprised by my husband. It's not terribly unusual, I hear. Midlife is a time when men and women often shift roles—men become more social and relationship-oriented, and women become more adventurous about being in the world.

I love being part of that dance.

Questions for Reflection:

1. When was the last time you did something different, just for the experience of it and not to excel? Think about things like dancing, yoga, pottery, art, or creative writing lessons.

2. Collect catalogs from your local college continuing education office. Highlight things that interest you.

3. Consider asking your spouse or partner to join you in the adventure.

# Chapter 21: Sweet Melancholy

"I love the word 'melancholy,'" my friend Susan said recently. "It's so much more descriptive than 'depression.' And it speaks so much to the soul."

I agree with her. When I hear depression, I think of an illness—something that needs to be treated or cured.

Melancholy holds a different meaning. The Greeks and the Elizabethans defined *melancholia* as an excess of black bile that produced heaviness in the system, and the condition was rather fashionable among the ultra-refined. People who were melancholy were considered to be artistic or poetic souls, more attuned to beauty and depth of meaning than were ordinary folk. I think of Elizabeth Barrett Browning or Emily Dickinson. Today such reclusive and gentle spirits might be whisked off to therapists and immediately given a prescription for Prozac. Their "social phobias" would perhaps be cured—but the world would miss out on some poetry.

Depressed people often feel melancholy, so it's easy to confuse the two states. But depressed people also suffer with what we call "vegetative" symptoms that can be deadly. Suicidal feelings. Preoccupation with death. Insomnia. Disturbed appetite. Severe weight loss or gain. Pervasive feelings of helplessness, hopelessness, or guilt. Difficulty concentrating. Lack of energy. Therapists know that to struggle with five or more of those symptoms for a period of two weeks or more is to suffer with a serious illness.

Susan adds another crucial item to the list. "It's all of those things," she says. "But for me the terrible paralyzing sense of *numbness* was the worst thing about my depression. It wasn't that I wanted to die. It was that I didn't care if I lived or died."

Many people suffer from depression—it's considered the common cold of mental illness—but Susan has learned from her bout with illness in a way most people don't. She has learned about her unique biochemistry and the medications that maintain her health. And, more importantly, she knows about descending into the depths of darkness and finding the nuggets of gold that now illuminate her pathway.

History is replete with stories like Susan's, of descent and initiation. In the Greek myth, Persephone is abducted and ravished by Hades before she emerges, transfigured. Psyche is banished into the underworld and given impossible tasks to accomplish before she is released and transformed into a goddess. Sumerian mythology tells the tale of Inanna, whose descent into the underworld initiates her from a state of blind naiveté into a wisdom worthy of her reign as the Queen of Heaven and Earth. The acumen acquired by women who have made such a descent shines through their eyes as Crone presence—a full-bodied magnetism that only comes from having relinquished the compulsion to be youthful and unconscious in favor of the gifts of a richly savored life.

Initiated women know a secret not generally shared by the culture. We know that joy and sadness live side by side in the chambers of the heart as two aspects of the same reality. The young are ever-searching for the illusion of happiness—that state in which the ego feels satisfied and in charge. Mature people know that the things that make us happy are always shifting. Outward circumstances change—and the ego, like a spoiled child, is always restless, always demanding more, yet wanting safety and security.

Melancholy is a life stance that accepts the vicissitudes of changing fortunes with equanimity. It enters into life's fierce beauty, searing pain, bubbling joy, raucous hilarity, and biting irony without getting attached to sentimentality or cynicism. Melancholy knows that we are fully initiated into our alive-ness only through fully tasting the range of human experience. While depression is numbing, melancholy is enlivening. While depressed patients suffer from "anhedonia," a fancy word for the inability to enjoy anything, melancholy people can enter into the richness of good company, wonderful food, vivid colors, vibrant music, and delicious smells. The state of melancholy, as Susan says, indeed speaks to the soul.

I've learned that the difference between despair and wisdom is often found in knowing when to retreat into solitude and when to seek the solace of community. I've learned that there are times when I need to be alone in order to know my own soul—but that the *need* to be alone shouldn't be confused with a brittle determination to "go it alone," or to forget that my health depends just as much on interdependence with a group of cherished friends as it does on my ability to be self-sufficient. And I've learned, too, to know that when depression or fatigue ravages my psychic life, I can be restored through a number of healing disciplines.

And as I gather with other midlife women, my soul quickens when someone like Susan articulates an essential and life-giving truth.

Questions for Reflection:

1. Notice the times when you feel melancholy or blue. Are your moods related to hormone fluctuations? Fatigue? Relationship conflicts?

2. Is there a part of you that believes you don't deserve to feel well? If you have any of the symptoms of depression listed above, see your health care practitioner and explore options for treatment.

3. If your moods simply ebb and flow, arrange to honor the fluctuations in your mood and energy by taking a mental health day or a mini-sabbatical, or simplifying your schedule during your down times.

## Chapter 22: Pleading Guilty

When you make a commitment to a new way of life, there are always unexpected obstacles. There are also unexpected sacrifices. A little while back, I brazenly announced that I was ready to give up worrying. I forgot about the power of guilt.

Guilt can be a useful signal. When we are thoughtless or careless or self-absorbed, when we confuse our self-interests with the interests of others, a tinge of guilt can remind us that we belong to a higher order or things, and cue us into right action. But true guilt—the useful kind— takes up very little space in the psyches of most people I know. True guilt can lead to restitution and healing.

False guilt is a different animal.

False guilt is worry-fuel. It's the busy voice that chatters accusations in the night. What we "should" feel or "could" have done. False guilt accuses us of yesterday's sins, for a past that can't be re-lived. False guilt never speaks of a today or tomorrow that offers us freedom and choice. False guilt hates freedom— because, every time we act freely, we risk offending someone. And false guilt is an approval junkie.

When we were young, we depended on approval. We needed it from parents, from teachers, from peers in order to keep the terror of abandonment or social isolation at bay. Authority for our well-being was truly in the hands of others.

Our task in midlife is to fire the authority figures in which we have vested such power. Psychologists call it a shift in the "locus of control." Our task is to claim our right to set our own standards and to choose the people with whom we share our lives. Most midlife pain is caused by the inability to make this shift.

I had a professor in graduate school named Dr. Polansky. He was a short bald guy with a New York accent and huge, sad, pale-blue eyes. He talked with his hands and he always wore a rumpled suit. He had a dry sense of humor, and he had forgotten more wisdom than most people acquire in a lifetime. His class started at 8 a.m. sharp, but I was always early. He said lots of pithy things. My favorite was, "Most people go through life pleading guilty to the wrong crimes."

I've played with that statement for a number of years, extracting different degrees of meaning, but what it boils down to seems to be this: As long as we accuse ourselves of false crimes, we avoid taking responsibility for real ones.

I talked with an agonized woman some time ago. She had been charged with a crime that stood to destroy her career, and she was racked with shame about it. Lots of people in her situation make excuses or deny their culpability—but not this woman. She was as awash with self-recrimination as anyone I've ever seen. Hollow-eyed with sleeplessness, she pronounced her own sentence. "People like me should just get out of the way so the decent people in the world can get on with their lives."

*Daphne Stevens*

I had been listening to her for a full hour, but I had to stop her there. "Now wait," I said. "The offense you have committed is serious, and there are likely to be big consequences. But I want you to talk for a minute about the woman who did this thing. If you were talking to me about someone else, how would you describe this person?"

"She was much too busy. She was exhausted. She was available to her customers 24 hours a day. She thought she was indispensable. She over-estimated what she could get done and she made promises she couldn't keep. Then she got into trouble."

"So you're facing the consequences—serious ones—for a crime against society. But what you're describing—the 'crime beneath the crime—' is the way you abandoned yourself." Yes, she agreed, she had always driven herself far too hard. With good legal counsel, she courageously moved through the court process, accepting responsibility while staying specific about where her real wrongs had been. When I saw her later, she had a long process of restitution ahead of her, but she was tremendously relieved. She had color in her cheeks, and her eyes were bright with gratitude for the "small miracles" that were unfolding in her life. She is healing, I believe, through her own willingness to separate false guilt from real transgressions.

Most of us, thankfully, don't face this kind of pain. But we all have a huge invitation to live our lives more happily, more graciously, and more lovingly than we usually do—and, as I see it, the ultimate real crime is to decline that invitation. We abandon ourselves to overwork. We betray ourselves when a gift (of time or beauty or friendship) is offered to us. We say, "No thanks. I couldn't possibly. I don't deserve it. I'm on a time— or beauty or friendship— diet." We deprive other people of the opportunity to be loving and caring, just because we are over-attached to our own notions of humility.

"The wisdom to know the difference." I can't know what the author of the Serenity Prayer meant by that phrase. But I think it has something to do with the courage to separate false guilt from real guilt, and to sacrifice both on the altar of something larger. I think it has something to do with a kind of baby-bird tenderness toward ourselves—a quivering grace that both gives and receives with equal measures of kindness.

Questions for Reflection:

1. In your journal, list the things you feel guilty about—"sins of commission" as well as "sins of omission." Where in your life have you hurt someone else or broken a law or a promise? Where have you failed to live up to your own self-expectations in a way that continues to trouble you?

2. Are there specific acts of restitution that seem appropriate?

3. If you feel called, make amends. Write a letter to the person you have hurt. Make arrangements to repay an old debt. Go to confession if that is part of your religious tradition. Or talk to a trusted friend to decide a course of action.

4. Now, go back to your list. Take action to forgive yourself for anything that rings of false guilt—incidents from your childhood perhaps,

or more recent events over which you had no control. To release the false guilt, you may want to see an energy healer or an acupuncturist, ask for prayer from a friend, or do some work with a therapist.

5. As you ponder on all of this, ask: What lesson have I learned about myself from each mistake I have made? These lessons are the mark of maturity and wisdom.

# Chapter 23: Words Fail

"Excuse me—I'm having a senior moment." It's a trendy thing to say. It's always said with a bit of self-disparagement, an apology for not being able to immediately pull up a name or a date. It carries a tinge of fear and a hint of gallows humor.

I don't know about you, but I'm troubled by the trend. It concurs with an ageism that is rampant in our culture—and ageism, although less "sexy" than racism or gender bias, is pretty deadly stuff. It serves to keep us from valuing ourselves. It divides us into factions, and it blocks vital gifts from being shared.

Not that I'm criticizing those who make self-deprecating remarks. We're all the products of a zeitgeist that hinges its false economy on certain myths: Faster is always better. Productivity requires a breakneck pace. Talking is better than silence.

It is true that, as we grow older, our ways of thinking and talking change. We're more likely to experience the "tip-of-the-tongue" syndrome, where we temporarily lose access to a name or a fact that is well-known to us. The conventional wisdom is that this signals a slippage toward inevitable dementia. But there are more hopeful explanations that are just as plausible:

1. Older people, by virtue of sheer time, have usually experienced more psychological and emotional trauma than have most of their younger cohorts. Unhealed trauma compromises cognitive functioning. The

memory lapses attributed to age, in fact, can be due to Post Traumatic Stress Disorder or untreated depression.

2. Middle aged people are often prone to neglect their own health care in favor of attention to their young-adult children and their aging parents. Very treatable organic problems, such as hypothyroidism, chronic fatigue syndrome, fibromyalgia, and the normal symptoms of menopause, can play a role in cognitive difficulties. Self-neglect in the form of sleep starvation, fast-food nutrition, and lack of exercise also takes its toll.

3. When we are apprehensive, memory problems tend to get worse—and Alzheimer's is an ever-present worry for lots of middle aged people. If we immediately diagnose ourselves with dementia every time we forget a name or overlook an appointment, fear breeds more fear and we become even more debilitated.

I once knew an elderly psychiatrist who was a bit bewildered by the world. Managed care and computerized record-keeping and even touch-tone phones were sources of frustration and confusion. He couldn't remember names very well. But his gifts to me were far more valuable than any recall of facts could have been. This man had well-honed instincts and razor-sharp insight and knowledge of philosophy and medicine and story-telling that often made a difference in whether or not a patient got better. He also had a keen sense of humor about everything, including his own memory lapses and his feeling of being orphaned in a fast-moving world. ("I feel like the bastard at the family reunion!" I frequently heard him say.) I'm thankful for the hours I spent in staff meetings where his wit presided. I loved hearing his stories about the old days, because he had been among the first to be trained in the then-new field of psychiatry. If he had been apologetic about his "senior moments," I would have missed a great learning opportunity. I learned from this man that old age brings its own brand of wisdom—an intelligence far deeper than words.

In *The Seven Intrinsic Rights of Individuality: Reclaiming Your Developmental Birthright,* Dr. Cindy Carter has observed, "Words in general are relatively new to the story of human development. Evolution compassionately endowed us with words, a parting gift as we exited from a more concrete and sensual way interacting with each other. There was a time when 'being' was the universal language, when we paid exquisite attention to each other's essence to decipher their truth."

Midlife "senior moments" spur us to return to that state of paying exquisite attention.

So what am I suggesting? That we just write off the fears of aging or the looming possibility of dementia? No. But I wonder what would happen if, instead of being apologetic about our occasional lapses, we accepted them as cues to step further into our authority as elders. I wonder if our positive impact on the world would be enhanced if we said without equivocating, "I'm sorry. I was thinking of something else. I missed that last comment you made," or "I can't remember her name right now. I'll let you know when I think of it."

Limitations and finiteness are an unavoidable fact of life. But the difference between despair and hope sometimes shows up in the ability to let go. To honor the deeper kind of consciousness that comes as we mature— a spiritual consciousness that speaks in the language of symbol and image that makes us essentially human.

My friend Linda is the author of a textbook that is used in law schools throughout the country. Writing that book was a major ordeal, and while she was immersed in the project, her husband Dan was greatly supportive. When she presented him with the final manuscript, the acknowledgement page was touchingly simple. It said: "To Dan. Words fail."

As a tribute to a devoted husband, the simple words speak volumes. I sometimes repeat those words to myself as a mantra. "To God. Words fail."

When I carry that prayer in the palm of my hands, I always receive a gift.

Questions for Reflection:

1. Notice what happens when you or someone else experience the "tip-of-the-tongue" syndrome. Do you feel embarrassed? Apologetic?

2. Consider the possibility that, in these moments, you are entering into a deeper way of knowing. Feeling temporarily inadequate in a social situation is a small price to pay for initiation into a reality deeper than words.

3. Remind yourself and/or your peers, "You are beautiful and valuable just being yourself. You don't need to capture the moment in words all the time."

## Chapter 24: Playing Hooky

Last week I played hooky. I had gotten overscheduled and frantic, caught up in delusions of my own indispensability. I wasn't sleeping well. I'll take a break as soon as this project is over, I'd tell myself. I'll cut back on office hours during the midsummer lull. But the projects kept coming and the lull never hit. I became more depleted with each passing week.

It's humbling. I spend my life preaching the gospel of self-care, sane pacing, and balance—yet no one is more tempted than I am to over-commit without even realizing I am making that choice. I begin to feel resentful at such times: Who is running this life anyway? Who is this taskmaster, and how did she take the reins again? And then, of course, I realize that the slave-driver is none other than my own self-important ego.

In the past, I might have pushed myself into an asthmatic episode or thrown my back into a debilitating spasm. After all, when you're wheezing for breath or hobbling around in pain, you have a perfect out. But I'm getting too old for that kind of nonsense; last week, I simply cleared my calendar. It took some fancy foot-work to rearrange my appointments, and I had some apologies to make. But the bottom line is this: When I've worked too hard for too long, I begin to simply go through the motions. I can't work with integrity unless I'm fully present. And sometimes the soul has to declare a state of emergency, just the same as the body does.

I set down some limits for my retreat. I began with the decision to avoid reading anything related to work. My overactive brain would have used such material as fodder for ideas about new projects or for thinking about clients whose situations concern me. The point, I had to remind myself, was a kind of re-birth into my vocation. So poetry and Scripture would be my reading diet. But in order to slow down enough to be open to poetry, I first had to simply sit. I listened to meditation tapes—not words, but om sounds and music that could envelope me in a protective psychic cocoon.

In a perfect world, I would have skipped town with only a bathing suit and a couple of changes of clothes in tow. I would have settled into a beach-house, Anne Morrow Lindberg-style, and written profound meditations based on the day's gatherings of images: sunlight sparkling on the water, pelicans soaring overhead in a perfect "V," the intricate ruffling of water and sand around scallop shells in that way that only nature's artist can re-create every day. But I don't live in a perfect world. My brain was too fried with this year's work to organize itself around reservations or travel arrangements. I had to depend on my inner landscape—the memories of past retreats—to take me into a place of rejuvenation.

I try to make it to the beach every year. To walk the shoreline watching the subtle exchange between sea and sky reminds me of something essential. To hear the soothing roar of the ocean—to let its music echo through my waking and in my sleeping—brings me home to myself. I am always delighted anew by the stark fierce beauty of that place, and by my childlike wonder at the ways the wind and water and salt and earth swirl together, creating the healing, life-giving froth from whence we all were born.

Thomas Merton was once asked how he could give himself permission to go into the woods and listen to the rain—how he could retreat that way from the suffering in the world. His response has stuck with me throughout the course of a lifetime. Merton is said to have answered: "I believe that, unless *somebody* is in the woods listening to the rain all the time, the world simply can't go on."

When I am more evolved, I will go into the woods and to the sea more often, to listen to the sounds so that the world can go on. But this season I must rely on my memory. I recall all the journeys I have made to the beach (or the woods) and realize with a startled half-gasp: This miracle goes on, with or without my consciousness. What a gift to stop and listen again. What a gift to realize that the roll of the ocean waves lives in me— as vital and as intimate as my own breath.

We've had a lot of rain this summer. I've moved through it fast, going from place to place. I've been thankful for the intense green of an often dried-out time of year, but I hadn't stopped to listen much until last week.

As I slowly disengaged from the world, my parched soul began to drink in earth- sounds—of silence, of rain, of mourning doves, and of memories. I began once again to ease off to sleep, to dream deeply, and to wake up slowly to each new day.

Questions for Reflection:

1. What are the things that increase your capacity to "play hooky," to let go of the workaday world and enjoy life's simple pleasures? Consider your favorite books, a retreat at the beach or in the mountains, or the simple practice of a cup of tea enjoyed on the porch before the day begins.

2. How do you feel about letting go of the world—a sinful indulgence, a blissful fantasy, an unrealistic possibility, or a necessary part of your spiritual discipline?

3. Write in your journal. Create a time of respite. Write reminders on index cards and place them on your bathroom mirror or over your kitchen sink. "I am visiting this earth to enjoy its beauty," they might read. "I am beautiful, capable, and loveable." "I deserve a day off." View them as loving reminders from the voice of the Divine that lives in you.

# Chapter 25: Hot Flash

It's midsummer in the Deep South, and I'm smack dab in the middle of menopause. Not an entirely unpleasant experience, I'm finding, if you're blessed with a lifestyle that doesn't require sitting in endless close-quartered meetings dressed in suits and panty-hose.

I remember older women colleagues of days gone by when I worked in places with rigid dress codes. The periodic flush on their faces—an agonizing blend of hormones and embarrassment—and the loosening of collars and the shedding of sweaters, are all firmly etched in my memory. I heard the half-apologetic, "Is it just me, or is it hot in here?" with a mixture of compassion and dread. I didn't want to be an Older Woman. Older women were neurotic and anxious and controlling—or so the myth went. Older women were all washed up.

So here I am in the heat of the summer, hot-flashing like crazy, feeling both humbled and edified.

I feel oddly privileged to be coming of age in this era. Medical advances mean that I am far more likely than my mother and my grandmother were to live into a healthy and vital old age—and yet the world seems pretty insane. I'm sure Older Women have been saying this for generations, but today's stakes are higher and the pace is more furious. Our culture is precariously poised between old ways of thinking and a vital new consciousness. As much as we want to go back to the innocence of the 1950s, the enemy is no longer Out There. Today's real weapons of mass destruction are harbored within our souls.

So I'm thinking about hot flashes, both personal ones and collective ones. Hot flashes signal the shift from one era to another. A woman in menopause grieves the losses of youth so she can see new possibilities. The medical community might label my hot flashes as the sputtering-to-a stop of my reproductive system—but the Change is even more profound than that. In menopause we *do* look furtively in the mirror for the inevitable signs of aging. But we also experience surges of intensity—body heat and moods and visions and imaginings—that are similar to those we experienced at puberty. The world tells us that our lives are waning, but actually these surges signal just as much potential as did the rush of emotions, fantasies, and libido of our teens.

Our country, too, is in a kind of midlife crisis. We want to hang onto old romantic notions of ourselves as good guys, and to believe that our youthful idealism will prevail. Some of us split into factions: We liberals (or conservatives) are the *real* good guys. It's those other folks—those conservatives (or liberals) who are trying to destroy our way of living.

Midlife crisis is always like that. At first, we frantically hang onto old ego ideals. ("I'm okay. It's other people who are making me crazy and draining my energy. And if I find the right ways of talking and acting, I can stay young forever.") We might have an affair or end a bad marriage or change our career or our sexual preference. In the midst of the transformation, it's hard to tell when we're acting out and when we're moving more fully into the flow of our lives. And then, as maturity sets in, we find freedom and contentment by focusing on our own responses instead of seeking new lifestyles or trying to change other people.

Hot flashes signal a move into a mature kind of wisdom. As I look about me, I realize two things about those Older Women colleagues of my past: These surges of body heat *do* make us uncomfortable. And it *is* too hot in here, in a culture that doesn't quite know how to shed its old skin and move into a new era.

Midlife women know about shedding old skin to prepare for new life. It's a cycle we have experienced for years. We need periods of hibernation and incubation—time set aside to rest and to honor the rhythms of our bodies— to remember what we know.

Questions for Reflections:

1. What are your associations with hot flashes and other menopausal symptoms? What do you remember your mother or your aunt saying about them—if anything?

2. How do these messages from your past affect you today? Do you think of menopause as a time of illness? of growth? of increased freedom?

3. Take measures to reduce the discomfort associated with hot flashes or other symptoms. Layer your clothing. Drink plenty of water. Take breaks during the day. Keep the temperature cool in your office or home. And abstain from any temptation to apologize for yourself or your

symptoms. They are a sign of your wisdom become manifest—of stepping into your rightful role as Wise Woman in the human tribe.

# Chapter 26: Money Talks

Some of our elders still live in the Great Depression. It doesn't matter how much wealth they've accumulated or how opulent their lifestyles have become. They live on the edge, always waiting for the other shoe to drop. Any experience of abundance is seen as a momentary glitch in a world where there isn't enough to go around.

Our generation has taken the opposite stance. Our prevailing myth about success was to have it all, without sacrifice or accommodation. Easy credit, glitzy advertising and internet shopping offered the illusion that we could have anything we want at any time—and that we should "go for it," no holds barred. The market is flooded with bestsellers about possibility thinking.

I'm fascinated by both points of view. Both are very much alive in me—the voice that says "Be careful. If you spend too freely, you'll end up as a bag lady," and the one that says, "Live for the moment. Think yourself rich. Do what you want, the wealth will follow."

Midlife beckons us to a third possibility. It asks that we relinquish both the scarcity thinking of our parents' generation and the magical seduction of Madison Avenue. It requires that we claim our own inner authority—that place within us where we trust our judgment while staying open to new information.

For most of us, income and outgo is a little like breathing. We feel expansive and we spend. Then we feel cautious and we focus on saving.

We sense a rhythm that allows us to spend when we choose, and to pull back without a sense of deprivation when it serves our long-term goals.

I've been thinking about retirement lately. I dream of time for gardening and traveling. I want to respect the needs of my aging body without a lot of anxiety about medical bills. And I want to live in dignity and peace, with a spirit of joy and generosity.

My desires are changing as I deepen into midlife. I remember my grandmother insisting, "I don't want Christmas presents this year," and I know now that she wasn't just being stoic. I, too, covet experiences much more than things. A festive dinner with friends or a trip to the beach with family, or an evening of poetry-reading doesn't gather any dust. It stays forever new in my memory, sustaining me when the days are long and I'm feeling discouraged or sad.

I don't think I'm unique in my thinking. What I do notice is that, while I can talk freely with my friends about health concerns, career worries, and problems with children and aging parents, there isn't much conversation about money.

Money is truly the last taboo. When people consult with me as a therapist, they usually don't balk at questions about sex. Those same people are pretty rattled by questions about their financial circumstances: How much do you make? What's your net worth? What's the value of your house? Those are the questions that send most people packing.

While I'm not a proponent of "getting it all out" as a panacea, I do have some ideas about this money taboo. For one thing, money problems send most people into survival panic, often the legacy of our Depression-haunted elders. For another, any problem with money— an accidental overdraft or a bankruptcy suit—brings up all-or-nothing thinking that gives rise to feelings of shame and incompetence.

The truth is that highly conscious, resourceful, and creative individuals get caught in dilemmas about money. When we lose sight of this, we miss a vital opportunity to know ourselves more fully: If I tell you my life story, you'll know something about how I want to see myself. If I share my financial history, you're likely to see a glimpse of what I hold the most sacred.

But how do we gain such self-knowledge? We're usually expected to just *know* about money. I don't remember a single course in personal or business finance throughout the course of my education. In my Southern family, the pervasive rule was "We just don't talk about money." And as a woman in this culture, I grew up believing that my fate was, in the words of Blanche DuBois, to "rely on the kindness of strangers," working hard, demanding little, and trusting that my goodness would be rewarded somehow.

Psychologist Anna Nemeth, author of *The Energy of Money*, has suggested that money is congealed energy—the measurable fruits of our time and our talents. I like that definition. It helps me to clarify how I'm valuing my time on the earth—where I choose to be generous as a conscious act, where I choose to bargain a bit harder out of respect for my gifts and my mission, where I take risks, and where I am cautious.

*Daphne Stevens*

Money is a road-map. It tells us a story about where we have been and where we want to go. It tells us what we long for and how our longings have changed and deepened throughout the course of our lives.

Questions for Reflection:

1. This week I invite you to look at your check register. As much as you can, put aside any notions about what should or could have been. Just peruse it with curiosity, as though you were looking at the records of a stranger you'd like to get to know better.

2. What do you notice about your values, your priorities, your passions and your circumstances, and about how you have both changed them and been shaped by their evolution? What story does your money tell you?

3. Are there any ways you feel moved to shift gears or to allocate funds for a neglected aspect of your life? If so, take it in simple steps. A small adjustment here and there is much more loving than an "austerity plan" that leaves you feeling deprived and impulsive.

# Chapter 27: Midlife Goddess

"I'm writing to you from a beautiful retreat overlooking a turquoise ocean," a friend emailed me yesterday. "I was reading your comments on Demeter and Persephone, but isn't there a story about Daphne?"

I was right there with her on retreat, gazing out to that azure sea. I was touched by the thought of her taking time to drop me a note. And of course there is a story about Daphne. I haven't looked at it in awhile, and I want to re-visit it. But for now I want to talk about midlife goddess-hood, in honor of my friend Margery.

This is the thing I love about goddesses: They're not stuck to any particular notion about who they are. They can be nasty and jealous pleasure-seekers like Aphrodite. They can be all-nurturing mothers like Demeter. They can be domestic angels like Hesta, or careerists like Athena. You put them all together and they make a complete woman. You keep them separated from one another, and they become stereotypes.

Who are the goddesses that inform your life? Most of us have known them intimately, one by one. Midlife is when we begin to put them all together—to enjoy the composite of all of our inner goddesses. To keep company with them. To be nasty and jealous without being afraid of being lost there. To be nurturing without giving ourselves totally away. To enjoy the exhilaration of a major career move without losing sight of other aspects of ourselves. As Jean Shinoda Bolen has suggested in *Goddesses* in *Older Women*, "By knowing who the goddesses are, women can become more conscious than they would otherwise be of the potentials within them that, once tapped, are sources of spirituality, wisdom, compassion, and action. When archetypes are activated, they energize us and give us a sense of meaning and authenticity."

I enjoy goddess-presence in a number of ways. I can strut around in a new dress without feeling vain—just quietly (or loudly) enjoying a visitation from Aphrodite, who, in addition to being nasty and jealous, is the goddess of beauty and pleasure. And when my daughter is opinionated, I don't judge her character; I see instead that Athena is present. It frees me up. Perhaps more important, it frees my daughter up. If she can fully experience her Athena-self, she will be able to know her other inner goddesses, too.

My daughter revealed some wisdom recently. She said, "When I was younger, I was preoccupied with the effect I had *on* people. Now, I'm more concerned with the connection I make *with* people." I pondered the comment. How many of us can make this distinction? How many times do I myself get caught up in "effect" at the expense of sacred moments when relationship is possible? I looked at my daughter with appreciative eyes. In such moments, the goddesses converge.

The story of Daphne is a simple one. When she is pursued by Apollo, she jumps into a river and is transformed into a laurel tree rather than submit to his advances.

My father was the one who named me. In my Raging Feminist days, I used to see that laurel tree as the symbol for my father's wish that I would never leave him—that he would see me turn into vegetation before he would relinquish me to any Apollos who might come courting. But the symbol of the tree has grown and changed as I have gotten older. This tree is rooted deep in the soil, right next to the river—the dream symbol of the unconscious. It is well-grounded yet it always reaches to the sky. And this particular tree is a laurel tree. A laurel branch is a symbol for peace and victory. I've come to appreciate the gift my father bestowed upon me when he gave me my name.

Goddess wisdom is like that. It tells us, layer upon layer, more and more about who we are. Its revelations unfold throughout our lives.

Questions for reflection:

1. What do you know about your name? What is its archaic meaning? How has the meaning of your name changed throughout your life as you have grown and come to know yourself better?

2. Who named you? What stories do you know about that naming? Is there anyone in your family who can enlighten you about that?

3. What goddesses have visited you as you have gone through the different stages of your life?

5. How do you see the presence of the goddesses reflected in the lives of women in your family and your circle of friends?

6. Have you ever changed your name? What was going on in your life when you did? What did you notice as a result of that decision?

## Chapter 28: Brain Building

"What do you do for a living?" a woman once asked me at a party. I can think of lots of ways to answer that question, but the truth is that I listen to people's stories. I've learned a great deal from listening. I've learned that getting older doesn't necessarily mean getting better, but it also doesn't have to mean a decline into senescence. It's much more complex than that.

Until the early 1970s, we thought people grew brain cells only until adolescence. We believed that after we passed through young adulthood, neurons began to die off, so that by middle age, we were finished.

In <u>Aging with Grace,</u> epidemiologist David Snowdon gave a different perspective.

Some years ago, a group of Minnesota nuns decided to give the world a unique gift. Retired schoolteachers ranging in age from 70 to 95, these women had spent their lives teaching and learning — and, along with Snowdon, they got curious about something: Is the mental decline associated with old age inevitable? Or can cognitive clarity be shaped and preserved by the ways we live our lives?

The nuns willed their bodies to science so that their brains could eventually be studied for posterity. They then committed to a daily discipline of doing things to stimulate their minds. They played bridge. They did crossword puzzles. They played chess. They read widely. Some took up gardening or learned to knit, or to paint or to work with clay. They listened for opportunities to learn new skills and to expand knowledge.

What we have learned from those nuns is astounding. As individuals from that group have died, scientists have examined the precious brain tissue that was their parting gift to the world. Even with physical evidence of Alzheimer's Disease, many of these women do not show signs of dementia. New neurons are created, it seems, even into old age.

I was gratified to hear about Snowdon's work, but the truth is that I've learned the same lesson from my clients over the years. Older people who seek new experiences, who look for adventure, who never stop searching for truth, and who continually add to their repertoire of skills, tend to stay alive and energetic. Older people who look for a reason to laugh every single day but don't mind a good cry now and then, who continually widen their circle of family and friends, are happy and optimistic. They say things like, "I've done my best. It's not perfect, but it's the best I have to offer for today" instead of obsessing over getting things "right" the way younger people often do. They live with joy and vitality, even as they struggle with the inevitable losses, the aches and pains, and the hassles of aging.

I've gained other insights from my clients, too. I've learned how vital it is to share our stories with others. Our life experiences provide a wealth of wisdom, humor, and colorfulness to children and grandchildren—and in telling our stories, we may actually build new brain connections.

*Daphne Stevens*

  I've also learned this: It's crucial to listen to the stories of young people. My grandmother and grandfather lived a long way away when I was growing up, and I rarely visited them. But I wrote them regularly, and their listening mattered. I couldn't wait to get those fat envelopes from my grandmother responding to all the news I reported. In listening to young people, we provide positive mirroring. We help them to make meaning out of their lives. We help them to learn—and, as they make connections and hone the art of expressing themselves, we grow in our ability to hear and appreciate.

  I've learned, too, that old age can be the richest time of learning in the entire life span. My mother-in-law, who died at 86, sometimes quipped, "Old age is not for sissies." She never seemed to stop learning. Even as illness overcame her, she read widely, she played bridge, she went to movies and to plays when she felt well enough—and she stayed connected with a variety of friends of all ages.

  Some of my best role models are the women in my water aerobics class. I love being with elders who enjoy the pleasure of slithering around in the water and swapping stories and comparing notes on the latest books and films. My friend Hazel, an 80-year-old who looks to be in her mid-fifties, says, "I've been doing this for the past 30 years. It's the best thing you'll do for yourself all day." Over the last few years, I've seen Hazel face devastating loss, disease, and disappointment. I've seen her look tired, but I've never seen her look old or dull.

Who will you be in your old age? As a midlife woman, hold the image of a healthy, vital, joyous old woman—and rehearse for that life every day.

Questions for Reflection:

1. Imagine yourself as an old woman. Write a letter to yourself as you are now. Tell yourself what you (as an old woman) want your present self to know. Prepare to be surprised by what your older, wiser self reveals.

2. What things are you doing to preserve your life story? Photograph albums, journals, even calendars saved over the years will provide a sense of continuity for your children and your grandchildren.

3. Consider taking up a new hobby to build your brain's capacity to make connections. You might learn to play a musical instrument, take up knitting, or research a topic that impassions you. Challenge yourself just for the fun of it.

## Chapter 29: Clearing Clutter

Feng Shui experts judge a home by the ease of the energy flowing through it, and I think they are onto something. I don't know much about the particulars of Feng Shui. I know intuitively that the presence of running water soothes the psyche. I sense that natural elements like plants and wood and fire and stone enliven a room. But experts also know something that good housekeepers take for granted. They know that clutter—any kind of extraneous stuff that isn't functional or beautiful, that doesn't speak of the character of a house's inhabitants—simply collects stale energy.

I'm getting ready for company this week. My good friend Cindy is coming from California, and I've been doing remedial housework in preparation—dusting corners she will never notice, cleaning out drawers and culling the bookshelves in my study. I want my home to be orderly.

I'm not usually compulsive when it comes to hospitality. In certain moods I can dim the rheostat in the dining room, light the candles, and spritz lemon Pledge in the corners. Add some fresh flowers and put out some hoers d'oeuvres or take-out pizza and—voila!—instant party. It's not a Martha Stewart kind of approach. I don't bake for days or crochet doilies for the table, and the scrutinizing eye may notice a few wispy cobwebs. The success of my festivities is contingent on the presence of a circle of colorful and fun-loving friends, a collection of good music, and a spouse who is more organized than I am.

## Watercolor Bedroom

But I'm feeling more pensive in preparing for Cindy's visit. I want it to be a retreat for her. She'll enjoy crisp sheets and gardenia-scented potpourri. She'll appreciate a rosebud in a vase on her night-stand and a generous supply of Vita-Spa in a basket by the bath-tub. Cindy is a healer, a teacher of some stature, and it's an honor to create a welcoming nest for her. I've known my share of California hospitality in her home, and I love returning the favor.

For my part, I need a wide expanse of time to enjoy good conversation and the comfort of the deep, easy silences that always arise between us. And I need uncluttered space.

Preparing for company is a chance to clear clutter. As I view my home through the eyes of a guest, I see things that I miss when I'm benumbed by the rush of the daily routine. Do we really need the old sheets and towels we never use anymore, but that I've stored in the linen closet for years "just in case?" Do I want to keep my bookshelves occupied with old paperback novels and reference books from long-abandoned hobbies? Clearing clutter provides an occasion to sort out the essential from the non-essential. It invites me to cherish the things I love—reading snippets of poetry from old volumes before dusting them and placing them affectionately back on the shelf. It frees me, too, to share things that other might find useful.

Midlife is a time for clearing out space. It's a time for year-to-year decisions about what to keep and what to relinquish, about sorting the things that bring us pleasure from the things we've hung onto out of sheer force of habit. As I sort out my things, too, I think about life's other precious commodities—time and money and, in the words of the Book of Common Prayer, "this fragile earth, our island home." I consider more consciously what it means to be a good steward and to relish the gifts of an abundant life.

Taking stacks of freshly laundered linens to the Rescue Mission, delivering once-treasured books to the Friends of the Library, has become a kind of cleansing ritual. And, when I return to be met with the sight of my newly ordered shelves, I'm renewed and refreshed. I again take delight in my homecoming.

Questions for Reflection:

1. Walk through your home as if you were a guest. Where are the places that feel cluttered? Don't judge—just notice.

2. Reserve an hour, an afternoon, a day, or a weekend—whatever block of time is realistic for you. If you have trouble organizing, ask a friend to help you, or hire a professional organizer.

3. Put on some soothing (or energizing) music. Spend the allocated time on a *specified* task—don't let yourself get overwhelmed by doing too much at a time. Clear your desk or clean out a drawer. Cull your bookshelves or your linen closet.

4. Take items you're ready to part with to the Salvation Army or Good Will.

5. Come home and savor a cup of herbal tea, enjoying your sense of accomplishment.

# Chapter 30: Empty Nest

Our son moved away last month—his first venture out into the big world. We made the trip with him to help with the move. It's 421 miles away, about an eight-hour drive. Longer if you're driving a moving van or a Honda Civic chase-car without lumbar support. Shorter if you're about to say "good-bye—have a good life—don't forget to write" to your oldest son.

I don't say oldest son lightly. He is mine by marriage and by choice.

The marriage part was accomplished when his dad and I fell in love while Ari was in the midst of an adolescence too burdened with heartbreak. He'd watched his mother die a lingering death. He'd been an attentive older brother, a devoted son, a steady student, and a dependable worker at the museum where he spent his evenings and weekends. But he was a lost boy. His father's whirlwind romance a year after his mother's death, I'm sure, wasn't easy for him.

The "choice" part came over years of quiet conversation and awkward silences.

I first saw what my son-to-be was made of shortly after his father and I began courting. He wandered up the street and sat at my kitchen table one bright summer morning. I was pleasantly surprised to see him on my doorstep, yet I sensed the layers of feelings between us. I'd already begun to adore his father, but I remembered his mother. How could I presume to have a conversation with this young man, teetering on the edge of the grand adventure of life, who'd had his launching pad so cruelly ripped out from under him? Somewhat clumsily, I told him how much I had liked his mom. I acknowledged how hard this year must be for him, and how too-soon this romance between his father and me must seem. How do you bridge the chasm between a seventeen-year-old's need for grief and a forty-something-year old's need for passion without someone getting lost in the shuffle?

    I didn't have to work too hard at making connections. After a few awkward pauses, Ari looked earnestly into my eyes with a tenderness that I have come to cherish. "I do hate it," he acknowledged. "It's too soon. I miss my mother. But I've never seen my father happier—and that's what matters to me."

    Ari's dad, too, is a tender man. He has defined grace as how you respond in the face of the inevitable—how tall you stand, how real you stay, and how much of yourself you choose to reveal. I've learned a great deal from these two men as we've muddled through the work of becoming a family. I've learned that there are layers of love to be discovered, and that being a family by marriage and by choice can be as intricate and sweet as any blood ties anyone ever shared.

    Ari's dad has had a hard time with this empty-nest thing. We went to Toronto last week for a getaway, and we talked about Ari during a day's excursion to the Royal Ontario Museum. Ari would love this, we said. He had recently told us a story about two rough-hewn men who spent their lunch break walking through the museum where he worked.

*Watercolor Bedroom*

"They checked their hard hats at the door. They clomped through the gallery in their heavy work boots, and their grammar wasn't good. But they really *saw* the exhibit. They talked about the play of light and color in the paintings like two little kids seeing a rainbow for the first time." As Aaron and I walked through the Images of Salvation exhibit in Toronto, we tried to see each sculpture, each painting, through the eyes of Ari's art aficionados.

We drove through gorgeous Canadian wine country for a couple of days. It was a glorious trip, but we were pretty tuckered out as we settled into an overpriced room with a splendid view of Niagara Falls. I was settling my things into the posh bathroom when I heard Aaron catch his breath. "Come quick!" he exclaimed. I ran into the room to catch a glimpse of the most perfect rainbow I had ever seen, arched right over the Falls. In that astonishing moment, I sensed that Ari—and we—were going to be just fine.

Questions for Reflection:

1. All stepchildren suffer from grief and loss through the death or divorce of a parent. If you're a step-mom, consider the losses your stepchildren have experienced. You can't be a substitute parent or manufacture a connection, but make a conscious effort this week to do something thoughtful or supportive for your stepchild, without any expectation of being appreciated. Prepare a favorite dish, or spend time listening, or encourage your spouse to do something special with your stepchild while you do something else you enjoy.

2. If you have children who have left the nest, write them a note or send a clipping or a photograph. They will enjoy getting mail besides catalogs and bills.

3. If you have young adult children at home, make a point to spend some time alone with each one. Listen to their plans for the future. Make plans, if appropriate, to visit a college with them or to fill out applications for financial aid. Join with them in envisioning their goals and dreams.

## Chapter 31: Unfulfilled Hopes

One of the bittersweet facts of midlife is the realization that there are some dreams we won't fulfill. It can start as early as our mid-twenties when we know we'll never be an Olympic athlete. Or when we hit our late thirties and sense that the dewy-eyed sexiness of youth is past us. Or when we wake up in our forties one day with a vague sense of defeat, and know that the hope of having a child has eluded us. Such losses can leave us with bitterness about the things that might have been, or they can deepen us into the life that has been given.

How can unfulfilled hopes and dreams bless us? Psychotherapists know that the best way to heal painful childhood memories is through listening to what those memories want to say. "I want to hear the things that happened to you," I sometimes say to a struggling client. "But more than that, I want to know who you were back then. I want to invite that past-self into the room. I want to join you in honoring that child, in listening to her, and in giving her what she needs." Such therapy is geared toward the notion that the inner child is a living presence with a wisdom of its own to convey. When we can welcome that child and listen to her truth, our lives can be gifted profoundly.

Unfulfilled hopes are like childhood memories. They hold an energy of their own. We want to hear them: the Madonna, great with child, who lives within the psyche of the infertile woman; the acclaimed poet who haunts the dreams of the unpublished writer; the "belle of the ball" who will live forever in the consciousness of the would-be socialite. These inner images are just as vital as the outward social roles we carry in the world, and they can bless or curse us just as surely.

I query my clients about their unfulfilled hopes. What can this could-have-been image have to say about your essential truth—your talents, your yearnings, and the possibilities you carry within you?

When I do Inner Child work, I assure my client, "This child is a central part of you—and yet we don't want her driving the bus. We need to let her know that she is a welcome passenger in your life, but you don't want a five-year-old taking the wheel."

Unfulfilled hopes are a lot like that. As we grieve the lost hopes and might-have-been ideals, we connect with parts of ourselves we may have forgotten. We don't let lost dreams and dashed hopes drive the bus. We relinquish the luxury of making ego-driven judgments about success or failure. As we let go of our white-knuckled grip on literalistic truth, we step into the ever-unfolding possibilities of the Now.

In my youth, I was impassioned by the theatre. I painted sets and ran lights and stage-managed community productions. At seventeen, I spent a summer in an honors program for gifted students, studying drama to my heart's content, and when I went off to college I auditioned every chance I got. I adored every exhausting, heart-wrenching moment of it. I reveled in the parts I played, and I grieved the many auditions I lost. I loved the sensation of stage-dirt under my fingernails after rehearsing a fight scene, of nightly donning heavy rehearsal skirts and button-down shoes to prepare for period pieces—but I was not a success. I was a gifted character actress, but I was too wispy, tentative, and otherworldly to play the passionate parts I coveted.

Yet I carry that fervent young actress within me. If I looked back on my years in the theatre in success-or-failure terms, I'd miss her gifts. Her determination carried me into countless auditions where I bared my soul and learned to withstand disappointment and rejection. Her enthrallment with character and theme and ensemble led me into the passions that have fueled my work. Her ear for poetry allowed me to enter a world where great stories are told and re-told, to hear dialogue whose poignant truths feed my soul even now. <u>Death of a Salesman</u>. <u>The Miracle Worker</u>. <u>Blood Wedding</u>. <u>The Crucible.</u> I hear their echoes in my consulting room; because they resonate within me, I can step consciously into the drama with my clients. I, too, am a failed actress. I, too, am a would-be director. I am all of these characters—the ones I played and the ones I wanted to play. I find that the roles I wanted to play are the most valuable of all.

If we live in a pass-or-fail world, we miss moments of rich possibility. Searing griefs and crushing disappointments are funny-shaped packages waiting to be unwrapped, reminding us, not only of what might have been, but of who we are in our souls. Instead of holding ourselves tenderly, we judge: "Is this going to be on the test?" we ask dumbly, like high school sophomores in the presence of a great teacher.

In my office, I have a Degas print of ballet dancers entitled "The Rehearsal Onstage." I like the play of light and the images of dancers, and

I love the title of the piece. It serves as a reminder: The rehearsal *is* the performance. Our unfulfilled hopes are the dances we dance.

Some melancholy evenings, I pull out my lost hopes. I put an extra log in the fire and I listen to Puccini's great arias. I read old love-letters and look at old pictures. I consider past possibilities: the parts I never played, the poetry I never wrote, the man I never married, the accomplishments I never achieved. Such evenings, I know, could degenerate into maudlin self-pity, but they never do.

Because after such an evening, I emerge into the world, re-energized by all the things I could have been. My unfulfilled hopes awaken me. They quicken me to the colors of the sacred Now ahead.

Questions for Reflection:

1. Think of yourself at age eighteen or twenty or twenty-five. What were your most fervent hopes and dreams? Write them down.

2. Now, gather these images around you, not as signals of failure or loss, but as living presences that are with you now. What have you learned from yourself in each dream you pursued? What do your past dreams have to say about your life right now?

3. Nurture these images. If you dreamed of being an athlete, consider supporting your local team or creating time for field trips to your alma mater's games. If you longed to be a musician or a composer, splurge for tickets to the symphony or the opera. Your presence in the audience will be a vibrant gift to others.

# Chapter 32: Time Away

We Americans have some strange notions about work and recreation. Recreation is something you earn by working too hard. Vacation is something you take to get rested enough to return to joyless routine.

Vacation comes from the word "to vacate." It is etymologically related to words like "vacuum," "evacuate," and "vacuous." It is a hollow term, reflecting the need to escape from something. I much prefer the word "holiday."

Holiday honors a healthy balance between work and play. It has a similar dictionary definition to vacation, but its root is in the word "holy day," a time set aside for celebration, commemoration, communion, rest, and play. Holiday—a holy day—is a time when we reconnect with things that are both essentially human and exquisitely divine. Simple pleasures—a long walk, good food, a game of cards, the warmth of sunshine on our faces—enliven us to holy possibilities.

Hurry—that violence we commit against ourselves in the name of saving time—is the main difference between vacation and holiday. "What did you do on your vacation?" people ask. How many museums, restaurants, theme parks, clubs, theatres, racetracks, did you take in? On vacation we want to do it all. We trade in one brand of manic activity for another, and we wonder why, at the end of the trip, we feel cheated, more depleted than when we started out.

On holiday, we let ourselves slowly drop down into ourselves and our surroundings, shedding the layers of bulky thought-patterns as we shed the layers of our workaday clothes. We may feel a little anxious about leaving it all behind—the business, the household, even the conveniences of home. We may feel a little boredom, too. And then we begin to re-create, to re-member—to swim about in the luxury of leisure.

As the spirit of holiday envelopes us, we re-discover simple pleasures. We eat when we are hungry. We rest when we are tired. We make love in the middle of the day. Our dreams become rich and vivid, and, if we are lucky, we find ourselves falling back in love with nature, with our partner or our family, and with life for its own sake. We return to the mundane world energized, more healthy and whole, with the sound of the surf or the song of the river or the whisper of the countryside singing in our bones.

Vacation—to vacate. Holiday—to inhabit. Time away can bring us both. In unpacking our suitcases, we can discover that we've brought home a little more of ourselves than we knew about when we left. A little sustenance for the work that awaits us. A sense of the holy in everyday moments when we slow down enough to listen.

Questions for Reflection:

1. When was the last time you took a vacation? Look at your calendar, and reflect on how you felt during that time—relaxed, busy, meditative, frantic?

*Watercolor Bedroom*

2. Plan a real holiday within the next three months. Connect with nature and read some juicy novels. Explore a place you've never noticed before—a beach, a lake, a mountain retreat. Take your journal, and jot down bits of wisdom that come to you to strengthen you during times of stress.

*Daphne Stevens*

# Chapter 33: The Language of Complaint

They have been together for 57 years. "We're still not sure it's going to work out," he is fond of saying with a wink. I'm not sure it's a joke. For most of those years, I was their emissary—the go-between, the third leg of an unshakable structure that formed the foundation for my family.

As I child, I was beset by their mutual grievances. "He's so passive! He just looks the other way. How do you deal with a person like that?" Or he'd murmur conspiratorially, "Your mother's so *sensitive*." I'd squirm, frantic to say something or make a move that would somehow bring peace. That was before I knew the Secret.

It took two graduate degrees, umpteen years of therapy, one failed marriage, a subsequent happy marriage, and thirty years of practice as a therapist to learn the Secret. I'm a pretty slow learner, but once I get something (as the kids say), I usually get it pretty well.

What's the Secret? It's simple: For some people, love is spoken in the language of complaint. Outsiders may want to say, "If you're so unhappy, why don't you change something?" Those truth-tellers—especially children —are usually called trouble-makers. Sometimes they even go to great lengths to *be* trouble-makers. Like court jesters, they dance madly about the palace, distracting the King and Queen from any possible outbreak of war. They often do so at their own peril, getting in trouble in school or with the law or becoming ill or sometimes never quite growing up, but always dancing madly and foolishly in the service of something they don't quite understand.

But the Secret is that such sacrifice is extraneous. Couples committed to the language of complaint have pledged their troth to that pattern. They may even see it as a superior way of communicating, scoffing at sentimentality or admonishing others to "get in the real world." One such husband, a long-ago client, insisted with a self-righteous snort, "We just say out loud what other people think about. At least we're direct with each other!" Like that's a virtue? I thought to myself. To just say what comes to mind without courtesy, consideration, or decorum? It sounds like bad manners to me—but it's all a part of the Secret, too.

Some people live in a harsh world that requires a simmering cynicism tempered by occasional bursts of romantic idealism. Christmas, for example, can be a time of great generosity. Birthdays can be idyllic. It's as though, for that one magic time of the year, a wife can say to a husband, "All that mean-spirited stuff—it's just a cover for how afraid I am of being hurt," and a husband can say, "I know that." And the spell is sustained through the opening of gifts or the dancing of the anniversary dance. And then, with the stroke of midnight, the spell is broken. "Truce is over!" they seem to exclaim. "We're not really that sappy! We're above all that!" And they revert back to the agreed-upon common vernacular—the Language of Complaint. They might even fight over the credit card bills incurred during the outpouring of mutual charity. "I only bought that because you nagged me about it for so long," he'll say, "There's no pleasing you," she'll say. Unknowing outsiders might consider that the holiday was a failure or that the generous gifts were insincere— but fifty years of observing such patterns has convinced me that, in some marriages, such shifts are no more significant than a swing from the back-basic into the promenade step when sure-footed dancers do the Fox Trot.

I used to get impatient with it. When a conflictual couple consulted with me, I'd witness a half hour of their mutual insults, and then I'd sometimes say, "You know, in some wedding ceremonies, the vows might be spoken, 'I take you _____ to be my lawfully wedded\_\_\_ _____. To love, to cherish, to honor and obey. To blame for every form of adversity that might come our way. To torment endlessly with mindless carping. To criticize and to deride. As long as we both shall live.' Maybe you should renew your vows."

Of course they'd look at me like I had lost my mind. I wanted to say, "There's a better way." They wanted to say, "This is *our* way." Through the course of the years, I got bored and irritated with the effort of listening—but I also came to respect the integrity that underpins those kinds of contracts. I came, too, to respect the funny kind of glue that held my own family together.

She slips away a little more each day into her world, losing track of words and names and the details that have colored their lives together. He cares for her as tenderly as a newborn babe, from monitoring her medication and preparing their meals to taking her to the hairdresser and keeping up with her glasses. When his children suggest, "There has to be an easier way than this, Dad. You're getting exhausted. Why don't you consider other living arrangements?" he gets a little huffy. "Not while I'm on the planet," he says. "She loves this house." Change is painful for most of us, especially octogenarians. And change has never been their strong suit.

I took him in for cataract surgery this morning. I called her every few minutes from the doctor's office, partly to keep her posted on his progress, and partly to keep her company. "He's out of surgery," I was finally able to report. "We'll be headed home soon."

The relief in her voice was palpable. As we pulled up the long driveway, I could see her in the distance, standing on the patio, hands on hips. "Who's that old woman in the red dress?" my father called out playfully. "Who's she looking for, anyway?"

As we ambled up the sidewalk, I saw a glimpse of who they might have been—perhaps even who they once were. She gazed up at him, flushed with the pleasure of his homecoming. She looked youthful and expectant and glad to see him. "You weren't worried, were you?" he teased her tenderly. I looked down at the ground, embarrassed and touched. Their naked devotion is part of their mystery.

I remembered all their near-brushes with death: His heart attack years ago. The high fever that led to her long hospitalization and diagnosis with this ugly disease called Alzheimer's. His broken hip and lengthy rehabilitation. Her carotid surgery. All benchmarks of growing old.

They are tender with one another at times like these. When they stand in the doorway of consciousness of their growing frailty, they seem to let down the veil. The language of complaint gives way to something more. I see something of the essence of their souls.

*Daphne Stevens*

My heart is full as I write this afternoon. I'm thinking of a photograph of a young soldier in the South Pacific a long time ago. He was handsome, my father, and as battle-weary as he looked, his face held an expectant energy not unlike the adoring welcome I saw in her face this morning. It must have been after their engagement, because I'll never forget the note on the back. "I know I look pretty old and beat up," he had penned in his neat block print. "But you made your bargain, woman, and here's who you're stuck with."

And stuck with him she has.

One of the gifts of midlife initiation is found in these places of seeing without having to understand. We often speak of the inevitable separation we make with our adult children. After years of pushing and pulling to get them to do things "our way," we find a liberation born of exhaustion and humility. We say, "Oh, I get it. It's not what I would have chosen—but it's not my life, after all. It's theirs."

Launching parents is a little like that. When we respect them enough to let go, we free ourselves as well.

Questions for Reflection:

1. Imagine a tableau of your family of origin, or draw a sketch or a picture of how you remember them. Did you ever feel caught in the middle? Did you ever try to "fix" any problems between them?

2. Now, imagine your parents with you outside of the picture. Just observe them and be curious. Let go of any anxiety you might have.

*Watercolor Bedroom*

3. Respect the integrity of their chosen relationship. How has any strength or conflict in their lives affected you? Are there hidden gifts or lessons behind any pain you might have felt?

4. If your parents are still living, call them or write them a note, with no agenda or expectations. Stay curious about your experience.

## Chapter 34: Parking Lot Sacraments

She's really more of an acquaintance than a friend.

We've greeted each other for years, at the gym, in church, across the aisle at the grocery store. Our gazes have met when serving communion to one another, in that otherworldly liturgical intimacy unique to Sundays and holy days: "The Blood of Christ. The Cup of salvation" is code-talk for, "I don't know the details of your life, but in this moment I see who you are."

But when I ran into her the other day in the parking lot after the service, something stopped me. Her large expressive eyes held pain—a quiet, contained, yet noticeable pain—and somehow the moment offered itself for real conversation.

We spoke of the silent agonies of midlife. We spoke of the terrors of having teenagers in the house—of worrying about their safety, of steeling ourselves against the onslaught of their ambivalence and hostility while staying emotionally available and vulnerable to them.

We spoke of the frustration and helplessness of watching parents age, of struggling with when to intervene, of the relentlessness of caring for them when they're sick, of holding the tension between honoring their dignity and respecting their growing limitations.

We spoke of the loneliness of gazing across the table or the pillow at our spouses during times when the only common link seems to be which kid we're the most worried about today, or which sick relative needs visiting tomorrow, or how we're going to juggle time and energy enough to meet the demands that press against us. And we spoke of the silent fears that middle-aged couples don't talk about: Is this all there is? What's happened to us? What will become of us? Will we ever connect with one another again?

My own experience says there is hope. My children, though still wobbly on their feet, are launched. My husband and I have nursed parents through illness and grieved lots of losses. We're not done yet—it's never really over until it's over—but we've moved through times that might have destroyed us. We're able to laugh about things we swore would never be funny.

My friend, in this moment, can't know any of this. She's still being blindsided by adolescent dramas. She feels inadequate and alone, and she's having a hard time keeping her footing. But just for a few minutes in the parking lot the other day, we shared secrets that will sustain us both.

In the Sumerian myth, when the goddess Inanna is in the underworld, her friend Eriskigal begs the gods to rescue her. Most of the gods refuse to help; only Enki, the god of water and wisdom, takes pity. He can't take time away from his godly duties, he says, to go to the underworld on a rescue mission—but he will do the next-best thing. He creates little creatures from the dirt under his fingernails. These tiny dirt-creatures will be his emissaries, he tells Eriskigal, to intervene for Inanna.

The dirt-creatures go to the underworld and bear witness to the suffering there. The Dark Queen holding Inanna hostage is so touched to be witnessed in her pain that she asks the little creatures what she can do in return.

"Just give us Inanna back, that's all." Thus Inanna is rescued. Through their compassion in the face of suffering, Inanna is restored to life.

Midlife women know this story in their bones. We have brought healing and restoration to others through simple listening throughout our lives. We have learned to do this through wiping away children's tears, writing notes of sympathy and encouragement, and caring for our loved ones when they are sick. We've learned to listen to ourselves, too, through a lifetime of movement in and out of the underworld, riding the waves of our own wild hormones. We are deepening into our wisdom now through the challenges that midlife brings.

But we forget about the power of our own quiet gifts.

We need to be reminded by stopping one another. In parking lots or in grocery stores or in churches or in gyms, we sustain one another in the journey. We become God's life-giving dirt-creatures for one another, and we deepen into our calling to be agents of strength and healing.

Questions for Reflection:

1. Have you ever felt sustained just by someone's willingness to witness your pain? Think about those who can listen without fixing, advising, or focusing on their own struggles.

2. If it's appropriate, make a gesture of gratitude. Send a brief note or an email acknowledging someone's help in your time of crisis. Light a

*Watercolor Bedroom*

candle or say a prayer in honor of the "dirt creatures" who have crossed your path.

    3. Be aware this week of small ways you serve others. Make eye contact. Offer a word of encouragement. Notice opportunities to heal by listening.

## Chapter 35: Sensible Shoes

They were simple pumps made of black patent leather. When I saw them in the JC Penney catalogue, I fell in love.

I was thirteen, and not very fashion-conscious. I was more at home in dungarees and sneakers than in the intricately-finished handmade dresses in which my mother had outfitted me since I was a little girl. It was, in fact, a huge bone of contention between us. "Don't you dare leave the neighborhood wearing those scruffy old jeans!" she'd warn when I was on my way out the door. "You go put on one of your Nice Dresses!"

"The neighborhood" was a loosely-defined geographical area, measured by who I was likely to see. It wouldn't do to run into somebody's well-to-do grandmother dressed in anything else but a cute little outfit.

In my fantasies I had always been a tomboy—no matter that I was terrible at sports. Tree-climbing had left me frozen with fear at an early age, clutching a topmost branch and waiting for my father to retrieve a ladder so he could rescue me like a paralyzed cat. I wanted to be a tomboy nonetheless—a horsewoman, a nature-lover, a camper, a swimmer. I thought the affectations of female adolescence were silly. I silently scoffed at the girls who giggled and primped on the school bus. I stuck my nose in a book at about age nine and didn't look up again.

Until I saw those black pumps. I saw myself dancing in them, feeling playful and feminine. It was in the days before panty-hose, so I saw myself in stockings and a garter belt with a flirty crinoline petticoat and a full skirt belted to show off my nubile waistline. In my fantasy I was the darling of the boys and the envy of the girls. My nose never got shiny and my hair never got frizzy. My slip never showed, and *no* young man would have dared to say anything crude. And anyway, if he had, I would have been charmingly dismissive, not rattled at all. "Ha ha," I'd laugh, as I looked down my un-shiny nose at any boy who dared to pop my bra strap at the seventh-grade social. I'd dance away with a boy *much* cuter than the Cro-Magnon who had dared to offend me.

The black pumps became a mission, a talisman of triumph in my newfound vision. The going rate back then for babysitters was $.35 per hour, and I worked like crazy all summer. In the early fall, I took the bus to Penney's, and beheld in person the black pumps that were to dance me out of the mundane world. My Cinderella slippers, delivered not by a handsome prince, but purchased with a jar filled with grubby dollar bills and shiny dimes and quarters.

The shoes were exquisite. The moment I put them on, my gawkiness was transformed into coltish grace. I didn't have much of a chest, that's true—I lived in fear of some boy looking down my blouse and finding me wanting. But I felt elegant and feminine in those shoes. I danced my way through the eighth-grade socials, still the introvert, still living with my nose in a book, but able during those magic evenings to allow those shoes to carry me away from anyone who might look at me too closely. In those shoes, I learned to love music with my body.

It's a crucial initiation for any woman, to learn to love music with her body. The inevitable self-consciousness of Not Doing it Right doesn't catch up until we're older—and if we've been blessed with a pair of good black dancing pumps and the imprint of a few appreciative glances, we can do a lot of healing as we come into our true feminine power.

I came to know later, of course, about the political incorrectness of all of this. No woman should have to look to a man to determine her self worth. I hated those pointy-toed high heels that came into fashion when I hit my late teens. The advice from the fashion magazines was "Don't wear shoes that are too uncomfortable. The tension will show up in your face." I read such advice with disdain, with the inner conviction that something was very wrong—but I pored over those articles anyway. Who wanted to be unattractive for any reason?

In my thirties and forties the quest for attractiveness gave way to the quest for comfort. When I became pregnant, I reveled in wearing "sensible shoes," and I never gave up the luxury of it. I wanted to feel at home in my feminine body. If they didn't provide heavenly arch support and sustain my freedom to move and to connect with the earth, I didn't even want to think about shoes.

"What's the big deal about women and shoes?" my husband queried the other night as we were watching television. It's true that we have a preoccupation with them. We're always looking for the right combination of sporty, sexy, comfortable, and stylish—but I think it goes beyond fashion-consciousness. Shoes, perhaps more than any other part of our wardrobes, tell the world about who we are. They shape the way we feel and move. And a good pair of shoes that molds to our feet over time comes to have its own soul (sole?) presence.

We in the West have an "I-It" relationship with possessions. We can't get enough things. But the truth is that everything we own tells a story about who we are.

Sometimes when I'm getting dressed, I allow my gaze to meander over the shoes in my closet. The hiking boots, the classic pumps, the well-worn sandals that I can't quite part with, the springy workout shoes, the holey old sneakers that are only good for gardening, and (yes) the several pair of dancing shoes with sueded soles for easy turns and glides. They tell me something about the terrain of my life—the places I travel for business and pleasure. They say something, too, about the state of my soul.

Questions for Reflection:

1. The next time you clean out your closet, re-consider the old rule, "If you haven't worn it in a year, get rid of it."

2. Regard each item in a meditative, loving manner. How has this dress or sweater or pair of shoes served you in the past? What places has it taken you? What story does it tell? Does it energize you when you wear it or even look at it in your closet? If it does, be thankful for its presence.

3. If it has outlived its purpose, bless it. As you take it to the Salvation Army or the consignment shop, say a prayer for the next person who will wear it.

# Chapter 36: Autumn's Kiss

As I stepped out for my walk this morning, the air felt subtly different. It was slightly cooler—not quite crisp, but without the mugginess that hangs over Georgia through Indian Summer. It won't be long before it's too chilly for shorts in the early mornings. I walked with a tad more spring in my step, savoring the anticipation of fall.

Autumn won't be here for awhile, of course. It will be in the 90s by noon today. Where I live, it's usually warm on Halloween. We get exhilarated about wearing long sleeves, and the first fire in the fireplace each year is cause for celebration. But this morning the first hint of fall in the air felt like the first ever-so-tentative kiss of a lover.

Today marks a special celebration at my church. The Episcopal tradition is rich in liturgy and pageantry, but we are short on initiation rites for young people. We baptize them as infants, we confirm them when they come of age, we marry them when they choose a life partner, but it's easy to imagine a kid getting lost in the shuffle between early childhood and young adulthood.

My particular parish is small but diverse. A woman named Judie noticed the need for a rite of passage for kids entering into adolescence. Lots of us notice things like that. We sit around in church or at the office and we say, "Somebody ought to do something about those kids," or "We really ought to organize this or that," but Judie just did something about it. She gathered nine kids together during the Sunday school hour for about a year. They talked. She listened. Somehow they all learned about taking on the mantle of young adulthood in a way that— knowing Judie— didn't feel stuffy or preachy at all. It probably just felt like having good conversation with a caring fun-loving mother figure.

So this morning those nine child/adults were recognized by the church. We threw a rehearsal dinner for them and their parents last night— just like a wedding rehearsal dinner, except there weren't any obnoxious relatives and nobody drank too much—in fact, nobody drank any alcohol at all. After a simple meal, we moved into the chapel, where the kids and their parents rehearsed the liturgy they would enact the next morning. Which brings me to the point of my story.

The priest, Dan Edwards, is a favorite friend of mine. I often quote him, and I love what he said to those kids on the eve of their initiation service. He told them about a scene from *Casa Blanca*, where Ingrid Bergman kisses Humphrey Bogart for the first time. Bogart, in inimitable Bogart style, stands looking startled and delighted and impassive all at the same time— and then he blurts out something dopey like: "Thank you." And Bergman, in inimitable Bergman style, replies softly: "It's better if you cooperate."

Dan looked into the shining faces of those nine young people. "Thus far you've hopefully been kissed by the Church. You will be kissed all your lives. But this is the time when you begin to cooperate. When you begin to find out who you are. When you begin to kiss back."

Hearing the words, I felt a thrill. I, too, was being initiated. What an honor to witness those earnest young faces, and to sense the sweep of time whispering through that ancient building. This, after all, is the place where my own infant daughter crawled in and out of the pews while I attended Thursday morning healing services almost a quarter of a century ago. This is the place where my grandson was baptized. I have attended weddings and funerals of countless friends here, and I have spent Christmas Eves and Easter Vigils and Maundy Thursdays in services that are always different, yet always the same. I have been midwifed through countless life transitions within these walls. It was in this chapel one Sunday that I gazed up at the cross and realized that the patriarchal language was too painful for my ears to bear. And it was to this same church some years later that I returned to a language much deeper than words, the blessing of sacrament, the comfort of hymns and chants that have come to sing through the cells of my being, and the largess of a welcoming community.

When my daughter was baptized, a friend said to me, "A christening is like a swimmer's kick. You can't determine the spiritual path of your children. You just give them a good solid wall to kick off of, so that, as they find their own path, they will know where they come from."

As a midlife woman, I am standing in the threshold of elder-hood just as these young people are teetering on the edge of adulthood. What I wish for them is this: I wish for them a sturdy wall so that their swimmer's kick can be strong and clear and clean. I want them to feel kissed—truly cherished—by their families and their community. And I hope that they will "kiss back," as Father Dan says, with passion and joyfulness and courage.

I came home today after the ceremony and studied my face in the mirror. It is different from the earnest young face that first entered the doors of St. Francis Church in the late 1970s. It is a face etched with laugh- lines and cry-lines. It is a face filled with its own brand of eagerness—and a passion that youth cannot know.

It is a face that has been kissed—ever so tentatively—by Autumn.

Questions for Reflection:

1. Did you experience a "swimmer's kick"—a religious tradition or a relationship that sent you on your spiritual path?

2. Where are the places that are sacred to you? What traditions have nurtured your spiritual development?

3. In what ways do you continue to honor those traditions?

4. Do you feel supported and affirmed on your path right now?

5. Consider acting in some small or large way to support the journey of a young person you know. Attend a baptism, a bat mitzvah, or a wedding. Offer to lead a Sunday school class or youth group for a session or two. Listen with genuine curiosity and warmth to questions or paths that might be divergent from your own.

## Chapter 37: Political Wife

My husband is running for political office. I love it and I hate it.

I love it that Aaron is involved in a dialogue that will shape our small community. Something in me swells with pride when I see him, gracious and articulate, daring to inject substance into public debates too often filled with boiler-plate rhetoric. I admire the way he challenges the status quo by introducing innovative ideas. It's a wondrous thing to see anyone unfurl his flag and share his gifts in community—but my husband is just plain dazzling.

And I'm exhausted. This election season has held me particularly spellbound. It's usually easy for me to eschew the morning papers in favor of an hour of meditation or writing or reflection on my dreams—but these days I am up before dawn, newspaper open to the editorial page before I am fully awake.

This race quickens me to the best and the worst in people. My husband's campaign has been clear and clean; mutual respect and good humor has marked his rapport with opponents. I've been touched, too, by the gestures of support and encouragement that have come out of unexpected corners. My husband is what is known in the South as a "two hanky gentleman"—the kind of man who doesn't feel fully dressed unless he carries not one handkerchief, but two, in case he encounters someone who needs one. He often rides his bike in lieu of driving, in the service of both his own health and that of the environment. "Why drive when I'm able-bodied and I've got a perfectly good bike?" he'll quip when it's 100 degrees outside and the rest of us are whining about having to get into our cars before the air conditioner gets cranked up. It's nice to see him acknowledged.

But the election has a darker side. Clean campaigns are too much of a rarity these days. I can't open my newspaper or turn on the television without subjecting myself to the attack ads that litter the political landscape. I'm exhausted with the adolescent mudslinging that permeates the airwaves and echoes in the gossip I hear around me. I'm dismayed, both by the mindless accusations themselves and by the righteous indignation they engender in me. It's arduous work, this business of being an Innocent Bystander.

Running for office means always having to have an agenda. I have spent a long time cultivating a life stance that has to do with being an observer. With showing up. With telling my truth. With staying awake. With letting go of outcome. The letting-go part is hard when you fervently want a loved one's desire to be fulfilled, and when you sense that a profoundly good thing is just this side of happening—and when you know, also, that vital questions are likely to be met with public indifference or cynicism or blind acquiescence to the status quo.

But I have learned a great deal this fall.

It began on a sleepy Sunday morning in August, just after my husband declared his candidacy. He had gotten up before dawn to set out on his bike to pick up some coffee and a newspaper. I was barely stirring when he arrived back home, smelling of clean sweat and morning air. I murmured sleepily, "Did you kiss any babies while you were out?" "No," he replied, mock defeat heavy in his voice, "The babies were all at home asleep." "Well, did you help any old ladies across the street?" I queried. "No," he responded with an air of dejection. "They were all at home, too." "Oh. So I guess it was a wasted trip." There was a pause. "But I did get coffee and a newspaper!" he added brightly. With that, we started our day.

That morning set the tone for a rich season for us. Playfulness weaves through a profound sense of purpose in our household. This race is the most important thing in the world. It is a call to public servanthood, the most sacred business on the planet—and at the same time, in the scheme of things, it is no big deal.

It's a dichotomy that is true of all good work, and one I have gotten to know intimately as we have ridden the waves of this political season.

Being in the political arena is an introvert's nightmare, no matter how humble the race. I hope he gets elected; by all rights he should. And yet the business of the Sunday morning rituals—the murmur of our voices laughing together softly before dawn—this is the substance of life.

Questions for Reflection:

1. In what ways do you see yourself championing a loved one's dream? It might be the financial concessions of seeing a child through college, or the time and energy required to help your spouse with a career challenge. List any situations that come to mind.

*Watercolor Bedroom*

2. Now, free associate the words and feelings that come up in connection with each situation. Does it feel like a sacrifice? A privilege? An adventure? Invite your psyche to reveal aspects of your experience that may be hidden to you.

3. Now, think about the champions in your own life—mentors or teachers who have taken great pleasure in witnessing the unfolding of your gifts. Write down their names also.

4. What about other champions in your life? Consider public figures, artists or authors who have inspired you.

5. Now, gather all of the people you have brought to mind around you in an imaginal circle—those people you champion, and those who have championed you. These are your psychic family. Draw a picture, make a collage, write a poem, or create an altar to honor them.

## Chapter 38: Strong Bones

My doctor furrowed his brow last spring as he studied the results of the bone density test. "You have a little thinning," he said. "Not enough to worry about, but more than we'd expect to see at your age. I think it's time for you to do some resistance training."

The news didn't surprise me. My grandmother, a great gardener who loved working long hours in the wind and sun, was stooped with arthritis and osteoporosis by the time she was in her fifties. My mother suffers from compression fractures in her back. She wasn't quite as physically active as my grandmother, but she took great pride in being out in the world, and it breaks my heart to see her largely housebound now. I definitely have the pedigree for "thinning," as my doctor euphemistically put it.

Yet I defied his advice. "Resistance training?" I quipped. "I've been in resistance training all my life. I get resistance from my children, from my clients, from my husband, and now from my parents. How much resistance does one person need before they develop strong bones?" I tend to make lame attempts at humor when my feet are in the stirrups, or when I'm faced with something I don't want to do. Besides, I've been devoted to exercise throughout my life. Isn't it enough that I've jumped around like a spastic marionette, flinging my limbs about and wheezing asthmatically in aerobics classes for the past twenty-five years?

*Watercolor Bedroom*

  I began to re-consider the doctor's advice when, recovering from surgery last fall, I realized how limited I was in upper body strength. And witnessing my mother's anguish—the pain it causes her to simply get up out of a chair— has left me helpless, wanting both to improve my own health, and to do something in honor of her suffering. Intercession for me often takes the form of exercise—I walk two miles on behalf of a friend who is grieving, and I swim laps the way other people say Hail Marys. I decided it was time to begin weight training.

  Two mornings a week now I meet at the gym with a personal trainer named Miriam. She puts me through my paces, challenging me to do things with weight machines and dumb bells and balance balls that I didn't think were possible. Miriam is a cheerleader and a midwife and a teacher in this process of strengthening my bones. "Okay, let me show you the correct form," she says, jumping easily onto a contraption that has to have been designed by Nazi war criminals. "Let's go for fifteen reps." She leaps off the machine and looks expectantly at me. I usually only hesitate for a half a second. After all, I'm paying this woman to get me in shape. She should know—shouldn't she?— what is too much and what is just enough. I enjoy the luxury of putting my busy mind on hold and just doing what I am told.

  I've surprised myself, these past few months. I find myself up at dawn, eager to get to the gym. Undiscovered muscle groups are making their presence known. "We're here!" they sing throughout the workout, and in the pleasant soreness that comes the day after. On alternate days, as I leave the gym after swimming laps, I find myself doing a few reps for good measure, just to assure myself of my growing strength.

Miriam uses a word that I love. Sometimes when I'm on the last repetition of the last set of one particular exercise, the muscle begins to involuntarily tremble. "That's great," she says. "You're working to the point of failure."

In weight-training, failure is a good thing. Failure means you've worked so hard that your body is saying, "Enough already! I give!" It means you haven't quite lost control of your form—you're not in danger of injuring yourself—but if you don't stop now, you might be overdoing it.

I like thinking of failure that way. I wonder how our lives might be different if we were to think about impending collapses and breakdowns as signals that we're working to the point of failure—the place of needing rest and respite. What if we were to simply stop, to pat ourselves on the back for doing our best, and take a break, instead of judging ourselves or pushing to the point of injury?

Resistance training is teaching me other things, too. It's impossible to think about your troubles when you're working a muscle at full capacity. And it's almost as impossible not to sail through the rest of the day when you're fueled by an endorphin high—that sense of well-being that comes from an hour of good clean sweat, followed by a bracing shower.

Strong bones, I hope, will be the reward for this discipline. But meanwhile the sense of intercessory exercise suffices very well. I pray for the women who have gone before me whose fragile bones were taxed beyond limit by backbreaking work. I pray for those who don't have the strength or the resources to move for the sheer joy of moving. And I pray in response to the sense of gratitude that pulses throughout my body.

Questions for Reflection:

1. Sit with your journal and jot down all the physical activities you ever remember doing simply for the joy of doing them. Maybe you played neighborhood kick-ball when you were ten. Or maybe you rode your bike to school, and you can still remember the wind in your face as you coasted down the long hill toward home in the afternoon. Maybe you excelled in school sports—or maybe you excelled in nothing except the joy of moving for the sake of moving. Invite that healthy, vigorous, lively girl back into your living space for a moment. What can she tell you about your life right now?

2. How would you rate your relationship with your body and your level of physical fitness right now? When you look at your list of physical activities, what do you see about how you might incorporate more activity into your life?

3. Do you see your physical fitness program as an expression of prayer and gratitude? How can you enhance a sense of incorporating the sacramental into your physical being—perhaps by wearing special workout clothes or developing a ritual around your workout time, or joining a group of like-minded people for a yoga session or a dance class or a bracing game of tennis?

# Chapter 39: The Essential No

"Just say no." It was the glib, easy slogan of the 80s. How simple. How complex. How impossible.

"No" was a brittle word. "It's a girl's job to say no," we were admonished in our teens. "Boys can't control their Animal Urges." In our twenties and thirties, sexual mores were very different—yet "no" still haunted our psychic agendas. We devoured books like *When I Say No, I Feel Guilty,* and *Don't Say Yes When You Want to Say No.* We attended workshops in droves. We wanted to be assertive—not pushy or aggressive, mind you—but powerful and successful. We memorized verbal techniques and body language the way faithful women of other generations have memorized responses to the catechism.

I slurped up the wisdom of the gurus. I, too, wanted to be assertive without being offensive— to learn the right moves and rehearse the right jargon in order to stand my ground. In retrospect, it was a rather simplistic revision of the social maneuvers I had learned in adolescence. "Always make a boy feel important. Ask him questions. Never focus attention on yourself" became "When you say no, do it in such a way that the other person— your friend or your spouse or your boss or whoever— feels affirmed. Remember to follow the Rules."

I grew up in an exquisitely chaotic-yet-somehow-genteel Southern family. My social training could have been lifted from the pages of *Gone with the Wind.* But a lifetime of listening to women's stories has shown me that my experience wasn't unique. Every woman in midlife today knows the Rules at some level of her being. How she defines herself in the world has everything to do with what sort of relationship she has made to the "Brittle No" embedded in those rules.

Some women, of course, acquiesce. They remain good girls forever, never questioning the social order, and living their lives in service to others. Unconscious and child-like, they never say No in any definable way. They often develop depression or physical symptoms. The Brittle No seems too brutal for these women, but their Yes is never really passionate or embodied.

Other women embrace the Brittle No. They define themselves early by acting out. They become enraged feminists or ego-driven careerists or intellectualized ideologues, and they don't feel they've really inhabited a place until they have planted a few opinions here and there. While the Good Girls find virtue in acquiescence, these Bad Girls feel that conflict is always more intelligent than tranquility.

I know these women because I have *been* these women. I've been Bad and I've been Good—and I've come to know something about life beyond both stances.

Midlife calls us to step into what I call the Essential No. It's a No that doesn't position itself in reference to notions about being right and being wrong. It's a No that doesn't convey rejection. It's a No that acknowledges what's given and what's not—yet it always stays curious, and open to the possibility of true relationship.

Most traditional religious teaching doesn't tell us much about the Essential No. We skip right over the part where Jesus withdrew from the disciples to pray, or when he declined to go to the side of his dying friend Lazarus. The popular question "What would Jesus do?" usually translates itself into a demand for self-sacrifice and indiscriminate giving. And while generosity is one of the fruits of mature, well-grounded spirituality, we can only be generous insofar as we say, "This is where I am located. From this soil I draw my nourishment. I cannot be uprooted without great peril to my life—and so it is here I will stay." That place where roots grow deep and healthy is the realm of the Essential No.

The Greek myth of Psyche reveals a lot about that place. Condemned by the jealous goddess Aphrodite, Psyche is given a series of tasks to accomplish in order to save her own life. The final task is the simplest and yet the most daunting. She is sent into the underworld to obtain a cask of Persephone's beauty ointment.

The journey itself is perilous, but Psyche's instructions are impossible. She is given two coins and two pieces of bread. Along the way, she is to reject the groping hand of a dying man who reaches up out of the water. She is to refuse to help a lame man. She is to decline to lend a hand to women who are weaving the fate of the world.

To give in to any of these pleas will condemn Psyche to the underworld. Unless she holds the coins in both of her hands, she won't be able to pay the ferryman who will bear her safely across the River Styx and back. Unless she keeps possession of the bread, she will have nothing with which to divert the three-headed monster who guards the entrance to hell. She will either stay focused and self-possessed, or she will surely die.

    Mature women know about wandering in Psyche's underworld. They've known the anguish of feeling stuck in hellacious marriages or exploitative jobs. They've been tormented by teenagers caught in self-destructive patterns, or aging parents who make impossible demands while refusing any real help. Midlife is a time when a woman either learns something about the Essential No or begins to slide into despair and bitterness.

    There are lots of paths into the realm of the Essential No. Spiritual direction and psychotherapy and Twelve Step groups offer companionship for the journey. Prayer and meditation and dream work and journaling are other forms of instruction. Reading widely and deeply— poetry and scripture, biography and story, and accounts from the desert fathers and mothers—is a discipline that many pursue. You will find your own pathways, and as you say Yes to sources of strength and healing, your Essential No will become more loving and clear.

    Your Essential No will bless and sustain you. It will teach you about the tasks at hand. Your no may be to an aspect of a relationship that you otherwise cherish. It may be to a job you've outgrown. A simple no may be in the act of turning off the TV, of limiting your use of the Internet, or of developing more discriminating habits in exercise or food or drink.

    The Essential No is a vital no. Through traveling its territory, we learn to sort the essential from the non-essential at this particular stage of our journey. Through the journey, we are freed to say a resounding "Yes" to a love much larger than ourselves.

Questions for Reflection:

1. Think about the things that cause you the most stress—relationships, job pressures, social or community obligations.

2. Consider the possibility that, in stressful situations, there is always a No that needs to be spoken. You might decline to participate in repetitive conversations that seem to have no resolution and leave you drained. You might resign from an organization that is no longer life-giving for you. You might consider a major life change that seems to be calling to you right now.

3. What support will you need to garner in order to make these "essential No's" manifest in your life? Consider drawing strength from your friends, your faith community, or a mentor. And don't forget to listen to your dreams. They are often our greatest sources of strength and wisdom.

# Chapter 40: Sponges and Mirrors

Sponges are much-maligned beings. We speak of "sponging" off of others. Being "spongy" has something to do with being wishy-washy, rubbery, leechy, or soggy. But it also has to do with being resilient, absorbent, porous, and springy—all those things we need to be in our youth in order to learn what we need to know.

I remember one day as a college student, when I realized I was a sponge. Biking from class to class on a perfect crisp autumn day, I realized with joy that my only job was to learn. For four years I had the pure luxury of attending classes, staying up late reading, writing, and contemplating. I was fortunate enough to have my tuition and basic living expenses paid by my parents. I was the original Goody-Two-Shoes—I didn't discover drinking beer and goofing off until later in my career—but I remember feeling incredibly lucky just to be a sponge.

This vocation lasted well into my twenties. I got gainfully employed and self-sufficient by the world's standards, but I continued to emulate others, wanting to absorb their wisdom, their charm, or their competence.

Being a sponge, when it goes on beyond its usefulness, is strenuous work. When you try to be a sponge beyond your time, you begin to be an algae-eater in the aquarium of life. You might find great role models to inspire you, but you also become a receptacle for other kinds of experiences. Overgrown sponges walk into a room, and with their intuitive, intelligent, almost psychic ability to absorb, they take on any anxieties, tensions, or worries that might be floating around. Sponges, at this stage, make great social workers. They pray for other people a lot. They hope that, by healing others, they will eventually earn a place in the world. And they basically drive themselves crazy.

I can't remember when I realized I was no longer called to be a sponge. It happened over time. Maybe I looked into the mirror one morning and realized I was no longer qualified to play ingénue roles. Maybe I got weighted down by the self-effacing sogginess that characterizes people who have overstayed their welcome in the sponge-world. Maybe it was the night I was walking on the beach and the unheralded thought came to me, "What if you're already as wise as you're ever going to get?" Or maybe a dream spoke to me and said in that unequivocal way that dreams sometimes speak: Okay. Sponge-days are over. It's time to be a mirror.

Becoming a mirror is a requirement in midlife, and mirrors are just as misunderstood as sponges. Mirrors are seen as the wicked stepmother's tool, the instrument of vanity, the symbol of narcissism. But a mirror can also be a good friend. And being a clear mirror is the greatest act of service we can offer the people we love.

The Aztecs have a story about accurate mirroring. It goes something like this:

*Watercolor Bedroom*

Quetzlcoatl was a great and immortal god, the creator of all things. His immortality was legendary, and it was well known that the only way that he could ever cease to be was by his own hand.

Tescodlypoca was a mortal god, whose name meant "smoky mirror." He was jealous of Quetzlcoatl, and schemed about how to bring about his downfall. After brooding over a plan for a very long time, he approached Quetzlcoatl and asked, "Quetzlcoatl, have you ever seen yourself as others see you?"

Quetzlcoatl was surprised at the question. "Why, no, I don't suppose I have."

Tescodlypoca expressed surprise. "How is it that you, knowing all things, have never seen yourself as others see you? Would you like me to help you?" "Of course," replied Quetzlcoatl. "Here. Look into my smoky mirror," offered Tescodlypoca.

When Quetzlcoatl looked into the distorted mirror, he saw a horrible, ugly dragon. He gasped and cried out, whereupon Tescodlypoca comforted him. "Don't worry; I can change how you look to others!" Tescodlypoca brought in great kettles of tar and helped Quetzlcoatl cover himself from head to toe. "Now, look into my smoky mirror!"

When he looked for the second time, Quetzlcoatl saw the horrible ugly dragon covered from head to toe in tar. He screamed out in anguish. "Please, I can't bear for others to see me this way. Help me!" "Of course," replied Tescodlypoca. He brought sacks filled with feathers and covered Quetzlcoatl's body from head to toe. "Now. Look into my smoky mirror so you can see yourself as others see you."

The third vision was even worse than the second. A horrible, ugly dragon, covered from head to toe with tar and feathers loomed in the mirror before the once-mighty god. Quetzlcoatl's pain was inconsolable. He raged, he sobbed. Tescodlypoca said, "Don't worry, I can help." He brought flask after flask of wine to numb the great god's anguish. Quetzlcoatl drank willingly. Finally, when he was no longer coherent or conscious, Tescodlypoca brought Quetzlcoatl's daughter into bed with him. Without any consciousness of his actions, Quetzlcoatl had sex with his own daughter.

Well, we can guess the end of the story. The next morning, when Quetzlcoatl awakened to find his daughter lying next to him, he realized what he had done. He was filled with pain and remorse so deep that he could no longer bear to go on living. He ended his life. That was the end of the Aztec empire.

I tell this story often, partly because I enjoy the way the names of the great Aztec gods roll off the tongue. (Try them: "Tess-code-ly-PO-ca" and "Kee-ze-CO-del.") They're just fun to say. But underneath the words is the message my friend Dr. Cindy Carter always adds: "Unless we know who we are, we live in great danger of becoming a smoky mirror to others, reflecting back a distorted vision of who they are. Only when we know who *we* are does our mirror become clear."

I would add this. The world is too full of smoky mirrors. Media-driven fantasies of perpetual youth and beauty are perfect examples.

Get-rich-quick schemes are others. You can probably think of personal instances where smoky mirrors are troublesome to you.

I became a sponge because I was in search of accurate mirroring—and it was an important and a worthy quest. But when we emulate others too much or too long, or try to absorb in lieu of reflecting, we betray ourselves and we overlook our gifts.

Questions for Reflection:

1. Where in your life have you been a sponge, drawing information and modeling from others? Where do you now serve as a mirror?

2. Who are the accurate mirrors in your life? What does it mean to keep your own mirror clear—to remember who you really are?

3. This week, be conscious of encounters that require each role. Note in your journal the gifts that are given in both.

# Chapter 41: The Third Woman

What kind of woman are you?

The question used to be a loaded one. Are you fast and loose? Virtuous and simple? Stylish or Frumpy? A Butterfly, or a Wallflower? In my youth, there were dozens of ways of categorizing myself. I'd rush to my mailbox every month to get the latest issue of *Seventeen* and take the self-help test *du jour*. ("What kind of perfume should you wear?" I once pondered endlessly over a questionnaire, trying to decide whether I was Woodsy or Floral.)

As we mature, we know that we're not so easily pegged—and yet, as I talk to midlife women, I hear the ways that we continue to struggle to know who we are.

What kind of woman are you? Do you experience yourself as youthful and energetic, or are you on a downhill slide toward senescence and death? Are you a Mother? A Career Woman? A Scholar? An Activist?

In my mid-thirties, I had a dream that I recorded in my journal as "The Third Woman." The first woman in the dream was coltish and high-spirited. Boundless in energy and enthusiasm, she was hopeful and idealistic and extraordinarily generous.

The second woman in the dream was quiet and radiant. Her energy was more subdued, and she exuded a peace and graciousness that would have been foreign to the younger woman. This woman gave of herself, but in a more deliberate, measured way. Great with child, her energies were devoted to nurturing the new life growing within her.

The third woman was less vivid at the time, but she was equally present. Luminescent and wise, self-contained and slightly fragile, she nurtured new life through treasuring her own wisdom, the fruit of a lifetime of walking with integrity. She gave of herself in less self-conscious ways, nurturing the dreams of those she encountered. And she knew something about the rhythms of life—about when to work and when to rest; about when to speak and when to trust the silence to speak its own truth; about when to give of herself and when to allow herself to be cherished by others.

One of the things I treasure about dreams is the way they continue to bestow their blessings through the course of years when we give them attention and reverence. Those three women still companion me as I deepen into the adventure of maturing and learning.

Sometimes I find myself re-visiting the First Woman. I want to be Youthful or Smart or Successful. I can easily let go of such formulaic labels—but it's harder to let go of deeply embedded social injunctions that there are right and wrong ways of going about life. I want to be as healthy as I can be, for example— but I feel confused by all the experts and their conflicting reports about exactly how to do that.

You probably know what I mean. You're living in your well-disciplined happy world, restricting your diet to complex carbs and getting your twenty minutes of cardiovascular exercise right on schedule, three to four times a week. You've made a well-informed decision about

Hormone Replacement Therapy, you're religious about mammograms, and you're reading all the right books. You're on the right track, right? NO! the experts tell you one day. Those complex carbs are turning to pure flab because it turns out that Dr. Atkins wasn't so crazy after all. Those cardiovascular sessions are compromising your joints, and your bones are turning to mush anyway because you should have been lifting weights all along. The Hormone Replacement Therapy that was supposed to protect you from heart attacks and strokes is now being shown to increase your risk. Sometimes I feel like Alice wandering through a Wonderland of Too Much Information, asking for directions. That Cheshire Cat keeps grinning enigmatically. "Oh, you can go this way. Or you can go that way. Or you can take the shortcut."

That's when I remember the Third Woman. The Third Woman knows there are no answers in this world—only questions. The Third Woman knows, as did the poet Rilke, that the juicy marrow can be sucked out of life only by living the questions themselves—by staying curious and open to new information, and at the same time letting go of the temptation to get too terribly anxious about any of it. The Third Woman knows that anxiety is at the heart of most human suffering—and that the compulsion to control the uncontrollable is at the heart of most anxiety.

I can't own the wisdom that the Third Woman holds for me. The truth is that I mostly invite her into my living space when I'm feeling discouraged or lonely. But when I get tired enough of trying to figure it out or get it right— when I can let the experts be the experts and let me be myself—I invite that Third Woman in. Sometimes it takes her awhile to believe that I really want to keep company with her ("Are you sure you're not too busy?" she seems to whisper). But eventually she always shows up.

The Third Woman knows what women have known throughout time. She knows about trusting the integrity of our healthy intentions. She knows that healing is not the same as curing—that we are all subject to the body's frailties, and also that our bodies are usually more resilient than we think. The Third Woman knows, too, that the "wrong" meal savored with a spirit of gratitude and joy can be more life-giving than the "right" meal choked down with a spirit of rigid self-control.

What kind of woman are you? Are you attached to roles and rules and types and categories? Or are you a woman who can host the whisperings of folly, of wisdom, of genius, and of vision that come to you in your dreams?

Questions for Reflections:

1. Consider yourself as a young girl/woman. What words would you use to describe yourself then?

2. If you have pictures of yourself, gather them together. Look at them as though you were an outside observer. What do you notice about the young person in those photographs—her facial expressions, her body language, her surroundings, her relationship with others. Is she hopeful? Energetic? Confident? Are there signs of sadness or tension?

3. Now, consider your "second woman" self—your early to mid-adulthood, perhaps the time you were raising children, or establishing

a career or devoting yourself to maintaining a household. What do you notice about that woman?

4. Finally, invite your "Third Woman" into your space—the wise future self who blesses you even now. What are the characteristics you associate with her?

5. In your journal, have a conversation with this Wise Woman. As though you were writing a script for a play, write a few sentences directed to her. Then pause, and listen for what she might want to say to you. You're likely to be quite comforted by her presence.

# Chapter 42: Silent Retreat

For most of my life, I've harbored a secret. I have been haunted by shoulds. It isn't easy to admit this. As a therapist, I'm in the privileged position of listening deeply and encouraging self-acceptance. For my clients, I personify confidence. But my own shadow looms large in the secret "shoulds" that whisper mean-spirited things to me when I'm not looking.

They started out early. "I should have been prettier," I thought as a child. "Then my mother would be proud of me." Or, "I should be smarter," when I received a bad grade. "Then I wouldn't feel so ashamed."

As I got older, I got angry. I projected the "shoulds" onto others. My mother should have been proud of me just the way I was. The teacher shouldn't have shamed me. While it's always helpful to know consciously where we've been hurt, the inner Victim can victimize us even more effectively than those people in our lives who have mistreated us or loved us imperfectly.

"Shoulds" are tricky little monsters. We think we are healed and self-actualized. We've gone through therapy. We've earned advanced degrees. We've accumulated impressive resumes. We've embraced the Inner Child and become Assertive and Powerful. I am Woman Hear Me Roar, and all that. And then we wake up one day and realize that our shoulds, like a bad virus, have morphed into a different form. They are dressed in different costumes. They might even show up looking like something benevolent. "I just want to learn from others and be open to self-improvement," they might whisper smugly. But they are still the same old Shoulds.

Shoulds always creep in subtly. "If I were a great teacher like Cindy," my should-monsters whisper, "I'd be doing something that really counts." Or: "If I were outgoing and bubbly like Sheryl, I'd be more successful in business." Or: "If I were creative and industrious like Lisa, I'd have written that book by now."

I have a circle of gifted friends, and there is probably a Should that goes along with each cherished companion. The truth is that I wish that I were all of those things—pretty, smart, outgoing, industrious. And the truth, too, is that I *am* all of those things. I'm just not perfect. The fatal poison of the Should monsters is that they always blind us to the beauty of who we are. They urge us to be larger than life, when being ourselves is really enough. It's more than enough. It's the greatest gift life can offer—a divine gift that is ours to claim as beloved children of God.

Last week I went on a silent retreat. For twenty-four hours, I marveled in the experience of being in the midst of nature, listening to a symphony of birds and crickets and other unidentified critters who sang to me from all directions. It's amazing how full of sounds the silence can be when we are sequestered from the electronic beeps of the world and fully at home in ourselves.

The retreat farm is a gracious place. A couple of humble buildings surrounded by South Georgia farmland. A simple room with a single bed and an open window. Meals, sumptuous in their simplicity, shared in silence. The sense of being welcomed and cared for, not for who you are in the world, but simply because you have shown up.

I sat in meditation the first afternoon, reveling in the realization that for the next twenty-four hours I had everything I could possibly need. I had glorious fall weather and woods and fields to walk in. I had my journal and some good hiking boots and a book of Rilke's poetry. Best of all, I had an expanse of time in which I didn't have to go anywhere or answer to anybody. Nobody was going to try to sell me anything. I wasn't going to have to have an agenda. I could have been happy just sitting on that porch savoring all that for about five years.

As I sat and walked and ate in silence, other things began to happen. Beloved friends and clients came to mind. As I was blessed and healed by the woods and fields surrounding the community, I became conscious of holding each loved one in my heart, resting in the certainty that God was holding them too.

The Shoulds showed up there, but they looked pretty silly—kind of anemic and sad, really. I'm not naïve enough to think they won't distract me again. But our demons lose power when we are in the right place at the right time. The right time and place has nothing to do with our position in the world. It has everything to do with finding our way into the silence and staying there until we can hear the tender voice that waits to sing to us there.

It's the crooning of the Mother. A Mother who delights in holding us in her arms and making up on-the-spot lullabies just for us. She sings in a thousand different languages and rhythms, like the infinite number of bird-songs in those woods: "You are my beloved child, and my favor rests on you."

Questions for Reflection:

1. When was the last time you gave yourself the gift of silence, for an hour or a day or a weekend or longer? This week, be conscious of the ways that the silence may be calling you.

2. Begin to explore options to nurture your time alone. Consider a visit to a monastery or a retreat farm. Spend some time walking, not just to exercise, but to listen to the voice of the Divine as it comes through the sounds of your breath, your footsteps, and the rustle of the wind in the trees.

# Chapter 43: The Difference between Men and Women

Agony was etched in my husband's face as he stirred from the anesthesia. I put my hand to his forehead—so pale, so cold!—and I whispered to the nurse, "Why is he in such pain?"

She gave me a knowing look. "*Men*," she said. "They just can't take it like women can. They like to be babied."

If I hadn't been preoccupied, I would have wanted to strangle the woman. How dare she make such an assumption? My husband is a decorated war veteran, for God's sake. I've seen him nearly sever a finger in a kitchen accident, neatly retrieve a tea-towel from a drawer, wrap his hand, tourniquet-style, and politely excuse himself to the next room before passing out so as not to disturb the dinner guests.

But—my ire aside—the experience of nursing my husband through this ordeal has convinced me that there are some unrecognized fundamental differences between men and women.

Take surgery, for example. When I found out I needed to have surgery last year, I went through the obligatory *mea culpas* about having to be out of commission for two weeks. I cleared my calendar. I arranged coverage for my classes. And then I quickly moved on to make preparations.

Two weeks of nothing to do except heal? It sounded like a stay in Club Heaven itself. Two weeks of lying around listening to nothing but my own thoughts? Yes, I could deal with that. I began to feather my nest in preparation. I bought cases of chicken noodle soup. I laid in supplies of paperback novels and cheesy women's magazines. I ordered healing tapes of classical music designed to synchronize heartbeat and lower blood pressure. I luxuriated in the anticipation of my own bad health. Two weeks to eat and sleep and not return one phone call? Not a bad deal at all.

My recovery was quick—almost too quick for my taste. After ten days, I was ready to be back out in the world. Ten days? But I signed on for a full two weeks! I went for early morning walks before I took my shower, and then called it a day. I had no illusions about being brave. I rested. I slept. I ate.

Men are different from women. It may have to do with being from Mars and Venus. It may have to do with our bodies being built for the rigors of pregnancy and childbirth. But I also think it has something to do with being willing to be needy, to be taken care of, to be—dare I say it? —puny.

My husband calibrated his recovery time like a mathematician. "Hmm. Surgery time. The average length of recovery. The expected level of pain." He might as well have had road maps and a travel itinerary.

He didn't get into the *spirit* of the thing. He was too concerned with being self-sufficient to be able to enjoy being sick. He was, it's true, half-psychotic on pain medication for the first three days of his recovery, so I can't fully hold him accountable. But he kept showing up in odd body-contortions—half in bed, half out of bed, determined to cook his own breakfast before he could even remember his name. I realized the man is insane.

In addition to being crazy, he's a big man. Our friends Beth and Donna showed up like angels of mercy. Donna is a physician, and Beth is a nurse practitioner who specializes in geriatric care, so they know about demented men who try to re-roof the house before they're fully out of the anesthesia. Beth volunteered to sit with Aaron for a couple of days the first week so that I could meet my appointments. "He's *tall*," she greeted me at the door after spending the first day with him. "And he's dense! You wouldn't believe how heavy he is just too look at him—he's so lanky."

"He's dense in more ways than one," I replied. "Did he try to reorganize the attic today, or were you able to keep him quiet?"

"No, but he spent a lot of time chasing the remote control. It kept disappearing under the covers. I think the cat is making off with it while he's asleep." Beth showed me a few of Tricks of the Trade—like how to get a 200 pound man out of bed. (First you turn him on his side. Then you have him grab you around the shoulders—not the neck—while you put your arms underneath his knees and swivel his legs toward the outside of the bed. Then you—hopefully with some cooperation from him—ease him up so that he is sitting on the side of the bed. Then you wait with him until you're both sufficiently recovered from that ordeal, to make the arduous trip to the bathroom. . .)

The worst moment in his recovery—the one that convinced me of the difference between men and women—was on the third night after surgery. For three days, Beth and I had both been ordering him not to get out of bed alone. I had left the closet light on in case I needed to help him up during the night. It had been my birthday that day, and as I crawled into bed, I prayed, "Please—for my birthday—just let me sleep through the night."

But it was not to be. Sometime in the wee hours, I felt the house shake. Before I was fully awake, I found myself sitting at my husband's side on the floor. He had gotten up, turned off the closet light, tripped over a chair, and fallen—hard. I quickly reviewed Beth's directions for getting him out of bed. Could I use the same maneuvers for getting him—and me—off the cold floor?

"Oh, no, I can do this," I heard him say. He was speaking in his Intelligence Officer's voice. He was back in the trenches of Viet Nam, solving an unsolvable problem, and determined to do it alone. I know that voice. There's no arguing with it. "Okay," I surrendered. "Do it yourself." This should be interesting to watch, I thought.

"All I have to do is grab this doorknob with one hand and grab the edge of this table with the other. Then I'll pull myself up and..." he paused, panting with the effort of it. "I can't do it."

It was the first time I had heard those words come out of my husband's mouth. I again reviewed Beth's directions. I ordered, "Grab me around my shoulders." In a slow-motion parody of a bizarre gymnastic act, we slowly got ourselves back into bed.

Now, I've been hearing about the Difference between Men and Women all my life. Is it intuition? Is it bravery? Is it obtuseness? Is it pain tolerance? But I've begun to know something more. Men think they have to do things alone. Women don't mind asking for help.

Is this a huge stereotypical statement? I don't think so. "It's a guy thing," I've heard from a number of men as they drove in circles refusing to ask for directions. It's a joke—and yet it's not a joke at all.

My husband is recovering well. The pain is finally subsiding, and he's getting back into normal life. We've both learned a lot. He's learned that he doesn't always have to be in charge. I've learned that I can take charge myself—I can insist on helping, even when he protests. We've become more aware of our interdependence and more tenderly appreciative of the ways that we do help eachother, every day of our lives. It's good to be needy. It's good to be strong.

Sometimes we can even be both.

Questions for Reflection:

1. Consider your own notions about being weak and strong. Do you attach any more value to one than the other?

2. Where are the relationships in which you can be both? Think about your spouse or your parents or your friends.

3. If you don't feel the freedom to be both, experiment this week with expanding your repertoire. It's very possible within the context of an adult relationship to say, "I feel like I'm about four years old right now. Will you hold me for awhile?" It's also possible in that same relationship to say, "I have to trust my instinct on this. Let's do this my way."

## Chapter 44: Giving Thanks

I've been reading a lot about resilient women lately. Stories of recovery from trauma, of triumph over oppression, of healing from illness, are everywhere. It's a significant trend, I think. The surge of books and articles and TV specials that focused on our wounds and our victim-hood seems to be giving way to something much more hopeful: Feminine strength.

As I write this, I think back to a day a long time ago. I had just gone through an excruciating divorce. My teenage daughter was acting out wildly. I was flat broke, depressed, and paralyzed by fear. I remember lying in my back yard, gazing up at a fierce and unyielding sky, clinging to a couple of clumps of grass as though I thought that would keep the earth from flinging me off into space.

My story isn't uncommon. At one time or another, our lives seem to collapse in on themselves. Major illness. Divorce. The death of a spouse or a child. Financial crisis. Someone recently asked me the question, "Why do some of us heal and thrive? What makes for a resilient woman?"

I think of my own resilience as a combination of dumb luck, God's grace, a few good friends, and the dogged determination to put one foot in front of the other, but the question is worth exploring. Having had the privilege of talking with hundreds of women has convinced me that an attitude of gratitude can mean a difference between emotional and spiritual resilience and the pervasive fatalistic depression that plagues so many people.

It's much deeper than the old injunction to think positively. I've never seen anyone pull themselves out of a real depression by virtue of positive thinking. But the capacity for gratitude is something we all share. Some are naturally better at it than others, but when we practice being grateful, we attune ourselves to hidden joys and pleasures that might otherwise get lost in the shuffle. When we literally count our blessings, we move out of victim-hood and claim our role as co-creator of our destiny.

People with a well-developed sense of gratitude enjoy a self-esteem that is lost to others. They appreciate themselves for their ability to learn from life's challenges. When things are going well, they celebrate the moment instead of steeling themselves for the day when things might fall apart. When things do fall apart, they know that all of life's troubles are passing events. Even the agonies of grief and loss become what the Christian mystics called "Wounds of Love—" transformative experiences that, over time, burn away extraneous baggage and bring us home to our essential selves.

Next week is Thanksgiving. I'll be gathering with my imperfect relatives to create a feast and share some stories and some laughter. I'll be particularly aware of those among us who are infirm, peculiar, unhappy, or otherwise too preoccupied to enjoy the present moment, and I'll notice those parts of myself, too, that are similarly afflicted. I'll be tired at the end of the day. I'll also be grateful.

A wise woman recently said, "It's important to know that, when we pray, we pray for the generations that have come before us, and for the generations that will follow us. In this way, we bless ourselves. We participate in the ongoing redemption of our families, in heaven and on earth." I don't think she means heaven as just an afterlife kind of thing. The Franciscan priest Richard Rohr has written, "It's heaven all the way to heaven. And it's hell all the way to hell. Not later, but now."

If the path to hell is paved with good intentions, the path to heaven is paved with gratitude. It's gratitude for the strength we haven't yet discovered in ourselves, for the friends we haven't yet met, for the moments of grace and abundance yet to be granted. We can't receive them if our arms aren't open.

Questions for Reflection:

1. This week, keep a gratitude journal. At the end of each day, simply list all the things for which you feel thankful. Don't forget to include the gifts wrapped in funny packaging—sometimes the things that hurt our egos have the potential to bless us the most.

2. Think of a time when you were in great pain, perhaps suffering from a significant loss. To what degree do you feel healed from that experience of grief? What did you learn about yourself?

3. If you don't feel sufficiently whole to count that time as a blessing, consider seeking the help of a therapist, a spiritual director, or a healer of another tradition.

# Chapter 45: Kitchen Work

It's the morning before Thanksgiving, and I'm in my kitchen. Chopping, simmering, stirring, and tasting are delicious prospects on a day like today. Transforming provisions into nourishment. Chatting with my children as they arrive home for the holidays. "Oh, it smells like dressing in here!" my son William greets me. I'm sautéing onions and celery in butter.

It's a recipe I clipped a few years ago from *Southern Living*. I made the cornbread days ago, complete with bacon drippings. Southern cooks don't worry about things like cholesterol count and body fat index, at least in holiday meal preparation. My grandmother used a recipe just like this one—or would have, had she consulted cookbooks at all. She was an old-school "dash of this and a dash of that" cook. She probably felt satisfied just to get a good meal to the table.

My mother made the holiday dressing after my grandmother departed this earth, but cooking is beyond her now. She's getting more disoriented. I get a call from my daughter, who is cleaning house for her grandparents. Grandma is scattering things, she says. She's pulling out all her recipe books. Grandpa is getting exhausted with it. I sigh. How can I do this without my mother feeling I'm usurping her job? How can I be here at the stove and also be there helping my father? It's not an unfamiliar feeling. Women struggle throughout their lives to be two or three places at once. I still ache when I remember leaving my toddler in daycare to show up at my job.

One of the blessings of midlife is the freedom to be in one place at a time— as Kim Boynton suggests in *Zen for Christians*, to greet each distraction as a friend, then hug it goodbye and take refuge in the present moment. I offer my daughter some words of support, and turn back to peeling sweet potatoes for the soufflé. I wish my daughter could be here right now—then, recognizing that as another distraction, I remember that I'll see her soon enough, and turn again to my peeling. I observe my own penchant for creating small commotions in my mind. Cooking requires that I focus on one thing at a time; otherwise I'm likely to leave out an essential ingredient or to carelessly nick a finger. It's good practice for me, this paying attention.

I'm imagining generations of women in kitchens, some with grim duty and others with a sense of generosity and abundance. It's alchemical magic, this kitchen work. Creating a bounty around which loved ones will gather. Do we know how holy our efforts are?

I'm not sure I've known it, in practice. I remember too well the relentless routine of throwing a meal in the crock pot before dawn, fixing breakfast and getting children off to school. I recall the evening rush from work to the table, the clatter of the family meal before clean-up and chores and homework— only to have it all begin again the next morning. This work may be holy, but it's also thankless, and I easily tire of it here in midlife; my husband handles most of the meals these days.

*Watercolor Bedroom*

But on a day like today, I remember how sweet it can be to inhabit the kitchen. My grandmother comes to mind again. She tended the home-fires, greeting us nightly with the welcoming fragrance of dinner—a platter of fried chicken and my favorite chocolate pie, or fresh corn bread and black-eyed peas. I recall the words of Brother Lawrence, and hope that my grandmother found comfort in her kitchen:

> The time of business does not with me differ from the time of prayer, and in the noise and clatter of my kitchen, while several persons are at the same time calling for different things, I possess God in as great tranquility as if I were upon my knees at the blessed sacrament.

I'm thinking about midlife and food. About being a woman in a culture of excess. About supersized fast foods in a too-busy world. I'm pondering, too, the irony of living in a country where women who starve themselves to be fashionably thin live across town from women who go hungry because they are poor.

It's all kitchen-work—this cross-flavoring of memories seasoned with insight. It's the alchemical process of turning base metal into gold, and wondering what the next chapter will bring.

Tomorrow, I hope my family raves over the dressing. But even if they don't, I will have been well fed.

Questions for Reflection:

1. Who did the cooking when you were growing up? What were your favorite meals? Food memories are sometimes our most evocative

ones, recalling us to times of feeling nurtured in special ways. Jot down some associations in your journal, and say a prayer for the ones who cooked for your family.

2. How do you experience your time in the kitchen now? What helps you find blessings in meal preparation? Lively show-tunes to keep you energized? Gregorian chants to help you stay centered? Special ingredients unique to your culture?

3. As you think of gifts for birthdays, holidays, weddings, or anniversaries, consider compiling a collection of favorite family recipes. You might include a comment or two under specific entries—memories of traditional meals that always included a particular concoction, the name of a relative or loved one who was fond of this particular dish, an anecdote about an occasion when the soufflé fell or you forgot to include an essential ingredient. Both the recipes and the stories can become part of your legacy to family and friends.

4. Remember, too, that kitchen work doesn't dictate that things be done in certain ways. This phase of life might call for simplifications you wouldn't have allowed yourself when you were younger. Takeout food and cookies from the bakery can be just as nourishing as the home-made stuff when they are shared with a spirit of warmth and celebration.

# Chapter 46: Anger Management

"**W**hat's wrong with me?" a woman asked recently. "I'm so angry all the time. I used to have the patience of Job, but since I hit my mid-forties, I get irritated at the least little thing."

"Did you always have the patience of Job?" I asked. I'm personally not sure that's such a good thing—but I was curious about what she would say. "No," she admitted. "Come to think of it, I was always pretty irritable when I got premenstrual. Now that I'm menopausal, I seem to have a chronic case of PMS."

This woman is doing what most women do when we get cantankerous or testy. We blame ourselves, pathologizing away one of the best measures of the state of our inner lives. "Anger management" is a commonly used term these days in mental health and legal circles. While learning to "manage" our anger instead of acting out of raw aggression, I'm afraid anger management gets equated with self-restraint.

Anger is like the gas gauge in your car. When your gauge reads "Empty," you don't smash it or judge it. You just know you need more fuel, and you stop at the nearest service station.

When our inner fuel tank—our reserve of energy and our capacity to give—runs low, we often get irritated. But instead of stopping for fuel in the form of good nutrition, support from friends, uplifting reading, or a good night's sleep, we blame ourselves for being on empty. It makes about as much sense as smashing that gauge in your car.

What do you do with your anger? Do you let it tell you that you're inadequate or bad? Do you hear it as a signal that you're getting tired or hungry, or that it's been too long since your last vacation? Do you honor it as a sign that you may be letting yourself be taken advantage of by other people? We can do lots of creative things with anger. One of my favorite options is to pray with it.

Yes, I said *pray* with it. Dr. Christiane Northrup, the guru of women's health, suggests that in menopause we undergo changes in the hypothalamus, the brain region that is crucial in the ability to experience anger. Changing levels of hormones actually make it possible for us to recall old memories, often accompanied by strong emotions, facilitating our ability to clear up old unfinished business. "Anger in women gets a bad rap unless that anger arises in the service of others," she says in *The Wisdom of Menopause*. In other words, it's okay to get furious if we are defending our children or harnessing energy on behalf of social justice—but to get irate because we feel used or violated is not in the script that has been pre-written for us.

Menopause is a time when we either let go of those scripts or we resign ourselves to walking around half alive in someone else's skin, simmering with soul-numbing resentment. Anger is a way of saying, "Get on with it, Woman. This is nonsense." It is an impetus to acknowledge our power—not for the purpose of control or revenge, but in the service of discovering who we really are underneath our assigned roles.

So what do I mean by praying with anger? When I talk to women who take their spiritual selves seriously, they often want to disregard their anger. I ask them some questions: Has someone let you down or failed to meet a commitment to you? Have you lost power, status, or respect? Do you feel insulted, undermined or diminished in any relationship? Have you felt threatened with physical or emotional pain? Have you had an important or pleasurable event postponed or canceled to accommodate someone else? Do you feel cheated out of something that should legitimately be yours?

Almost always, there is a dawning of recognition. "Well, yes, I'm always putting my own needs on hold to baby-sit my grandchildren/listen to a friend with a problem/work late for my boss/entertain my husband's colleagues." And almost always a qualifier is added: "But isn't that what a mother/wife/friend is supposed to do?"

Absolutely not. If you are accommodating other people enough to feel irritated or angry, you're running on empty—and that's a dangerous condition, right up there with hypertension and high cholesterol and obesity. And if your doctor were to advise you to change your lifestyle habits to correct one of those conditions, you probably wouldn't be saying, "But isn't a woman *supposed* to have high blood pressure?"

So this is what I mean by praying with anger. First, it's important to honor anger in the same way that we honor that gas gauge in our car—as a signal that something else is needed. It's a God-given warning sign, like pain when we're injured. After we identify what is needed, it's important to act. But in praying with our anger, we commit ourselves to action that is measured and fully considered. We sit with uncomfortable feelings. We knowledge the hurt that lies just beneath the surface. We may even move into a loving-kindness meditation in which we breathe in the anger and breathe out good will—but we don't try to spiritualize it away. We embrace the anger just as we would receive an unexpected guest, asking it what it wants to say to us. And when the time is right, we move into right action.

Right action in response to anger is a prayerful move. It differs from *re*action. We don't give away our power to anyone else with a "Look what you made me do!" attitude. We stay centered within ourselves to determine whether or not a confrontation is advisable. Do we want to invest our energy in an encounter with the person who has hurt us? Is it a wise use of our energy? Or do we need to acknowledge that the offending party is caught in a hurtful and destructive pattern and not worthy right now of too much honesty? Religious tradition calls this the gift of discernment, but I am amazed sometimes at the number of people who believe that their religious calling is to be doormats or control-freaks.

I personally need a lot of support in deciding right action in a charged situation. You might draw on the wisdom of a good friend or a therapist or a support group or a mentor to help you to map out a plan. The plan should be consistent with your values as well as your most realistic expectations.

Right action in response to anger is an important task for midlife women. Through right action, we differentiate ourselves from other people. We say, "This is where you end and I begin." We affirm our own right to exist on the planet, to need what we need and to want what we want. We find the courage to say, "There's enough to go around. I don't have to deny myself in order for others to get what they need." Through right action, we don't rehearse for more anger. We clear the air in a way that helps us see ourselves and others more lovingly—not the feel-good kind of love that says "Aren't I a nice person?" but the full-bodied love that sees all the way down to the bones of our shared human foibles.

Through praying our anger, we own our authority as elders of the human tribe. We relinquish the role of caretaking ingénue. We step up to the plate and tend the world's soul.

Questions for Reflection:

1. Think of someone with whom you are angry or irritated. Can you pinpoint the reason you are offended? Have you been let down or disappointed by something they've done? Have you felt put down or diminished by them? Have they harmed you either physically or emotionally? Articulate the nature of the offense, perhaps in your journal, or with a trusted friend.

2. Ask yourself, "What action is called for here?" (Remember that anger always calls for some response.) Perhaps you need to confront the person. Maybe you need to write a letter—you can decide later whether to mail it, but just get the anger off your chest for now. Perhaps you need to work through your feelings within the safety of a trusted container— with a priest or a therapist or a circle of friends. (You'll know you're working through the feelings and not just gossiping if the conversation releases you from the tyranny of anger).

3. Sit in silence or take a walk. If you can, practice a loving-kindness meditation, sending positive energy to the person who has offended you.

4. Recognize your role in tending the soul of the world through your creative response to a difficult situation.

# Chapter 47: The Long Road Toward Goodbye

Being middle-aged is easier than being old. When you're old, you face a frightening and uncertain future, without much empathy from the larger community. Your days are marked by reminding yourself to take your medications. To go to the doctor. To watch the TV shows that grant you contact with the outside world. You're plagued with aches and pains. Worst of all, you're likely to feel invisible.

I don't anticipate such a future for myself, of course. I hope to keep from losing my mind or my sight or my hearing, to enjoy a vital old age followed by a peaceful death.

But these are just hopes. I'm not old yet, just aging. And it's not my own aches and pains and isolation that worry me right now. I'm the daughter of elderly parents.

You probably know how it goes. You begin to notice that your mother is getting confused. She's always been absent-minded, so you ignore it at first. It's irritating, really, the way she repeats herself, the way she insists on dispensing advice about things she doesn't know about. You find yourself wanting to cut visits short. You feel slightly guilty as you pull out of the driveway, but remorse is tempered with annoyance. Hey, I've been there, you tell yourself. I've done the teenage thing with her. I've listened to endless admonitions, I've conformed to the pressure to meet her demands. I'm a grown-up now. You move back to your well-defined life.

But her confusion begins to get bizarre. Quirky habits that characterized her when she was younger—the compulsion to wash out plastic bags for re-use, the piles of newspapers and magazines she kept in the corner ("I'm too busy to read them now, but I'll get to them later. Don't throw them away!"), the stockpile of nightgowns with tags still on them bought on sale—begin to seem like obsessions.

She's getting frail. You know it. Your father calls regularly, always with a mixture of desperation and denial in his voice. "I hate to bother you," he says one Sunday morning, "but your mother is sick. I can't get her out of bed."

The drive to their house seems longer than usual, but you make it in record time. Her body is hot with a raging fever. She's talking out of her head. "How long has she been like this?" you ask. "About three days," your father says. "Have you called the doctor?" you ask. "No," he says. "I didn't want to be a nuisance."

Being a nuisance is the last thing you're worried about. "Call an ambulance and meet me in the emergency room," the doctor says. You make the call, then go into the kitchen. Your father is pulling things out of the freezer. "Won't you have lunch with us?" he asks. "We have a good pork roast and fried apples and macaroni."

After a long vigil in the Emergency Room, a foreign doctor comes in with the news. You are bleary eyed from the watching and waiting, and you can barely understand his broken English. She has a rare virus, he tells you. She'll need several days of IV antibiotics. Maybe she'll survive, maybe she won't. And, by the way, the X-rays have revealed a compression fracture in her back. .

The hospital stay is a roller-coaster ride. She's better one day and worse the next. You spend the night on a cot in her room, and your aching back reminds you in the morning that you, too, are not as young as you used to be. You offer her ice chips and small spoonfuls of jello. You rub her hands and feet with lotion. Sometimes she knows you and sometimes she doesn't.

When you're not with her, you're pacing the halls trying to keep up with your father. He's worried and anxious. You stop him and say, "Sit down, Dad. Let's rest a minute." You look into his eyes. This is a man who has worked hard all his life to provide for his family. He is the one who taught you to love poetry and classical music. You want to say, "You need a rest. Go home, Dad. I'll take care of things here." What comes out of your mouth is, "Did you and Mother ever sign durable-power-of-attorney-for-health-care?"

It's a conversation you've tried to have before, but the hurt in his eyes is worse than a slap. "That's the paperwork that has to do with pulling the plug, isn't it?"

Oh, Dad. It's the paperwork that keeps you in charge of your own affairs, and keeps your children from having to guess. You feel annoyed. He's savvy, he's smart. Why can't he focus for a moment on the business at hand? As you continue to look into his eyes, you realize that grief and fear are the only business that he can attend to.

You brush back a stray hair from his forehead. It feels like the end, but you sense it's only the beginning. "You need a rest. Go home, Dad. I'll take care of things for awhile."

Questions for Reflection:

1. Are there elderly people in your family for whom you feel responsible? Think of them—a parent, an aunt, or even a disabled sibling.

2. Visualize what you'd like to provide for them—the role you'd like to play in their lives. Write a few notes in your journal.

3. Now, in the context of your family life, what things are realistic for you to do? To invite them to move in with you? To arrange for a sitter or a caregiver? To visit them in a nursing home? Or none of the above? Remember that there are no right or wrong ways to walk through this phase of life. Your response is dependent on your family history, your own level of healing and growth, and your other responsibilities.

4. Take a concrete step toward care-giving if it's appropriate. Begin to gather the names of sitters. Call a brother or sister and express your concerns. Call your parents and express your appreciation for what they have done for you, or, if you live in the same town, offer to bring them lunch on a Sunday afternoon.

5. Now, practice letting go. See a movie, read a novel, or sit in your favorite coffee house with your journal.

6. Call a friend who is struggling with the care of an elderly parent, and offer a few words of encouragement. At this stage of life, we need our women friends more than ever. Lisa Groen Braner, in *The Mother's Book*

*of Well-Being*, has said of young motherhood, "It is a lot like running a marathon. You have to pace yourself, and you have to be in good condition to see the race through. You also need people handing you water along the way." How true this is in caring for elderly parents! We need to be caregivers to one another.

## Chapter 48: Accidental Joy

Bible scholars know about a quote "the day of the Lord will come like a thief in the night." I'm not a preacher or a Bible scholar, but at Christmastime that passage takes on a whole new meaning.

For me, Christmas comes like a thief in the night. I resist it like crazy all year long. My introverted self flinches at the thought of endless rounds of manic activity. My perfectionistic self goes into a spin at the prospect of finding appropriate gifts. I am troubled by a culture that devotes one season— one of the holiest seasons of the year— to consumerism and overeating. Yes, I admit it, I'm a Scrooge.

I've written countless articles for magazines and newspapers through the years: Christmas Blues and Holiday Stress and Seasonal Affective Disorder are all catchy topics. Everyone wants advice on dealing with holiday problems. How to cope with the friend who drinks too much, or the relatives who don't get along, or the kids who look expectantly for Santa Claus when the budget is already stretched beyond all reasonable limits? How to come to terms with our own sense of loss when faced with endless neediness and loneliness, sometimes within the circle of our own families? I write for my clients and my readers—but most of all, I write for myself. How do I keep my equilibrium and find a modicum of balance and meaning in a season whose main distinction is its too-muchness?

But somewhere in the course of December, a sense of joy always claims me. It mostly happens by accident. I see an acquaintance in the mall, and she hails me with a hearty greeting. In the midst of the noise and the pandemonium, I remember that her mother died this past year, or that she is in the middle of a divorce. Or we reminisce briefly about when our kids were in kindergarten together, and we marvel about how they're all grown up. In that moment of connection, an old truth reclaims me: The chaos, the confusion, the sense of inadequacy of the season are a microcosm of the world we live in—and joy always claims us in unexpected ways.

This year, accidental joy has come twice. In early December, I went with my friend Lucille to see a touring production of *Fosse*. The dancers were precise to the point of perfection, their undulating movements so beautiful that it almost hurt to watch. As we sat in the darkened theatre, I realized that Lucille was faintly humming along with the music— she was almost imperceptibly dancing in her seat. I smiled in the dark, relinquishing myself to the trance of the evening.

*Fosse* is an incredible show, but it is not what I call a happy one. Bob Fosse was one of the greatest choreographers of all time, but his genius was haunted by pathos and chaos. As I moved into the world of the play, I thought: This is Christmas. It's the chaos and the pathos—and it's the ecstasy of dancing just for the sake of dancing, and of sitting in the dark and seeing things that are almost too beautiful to bear.

A second moment of joy occurred this week. In Walgreen's waiting for a prescription to be filled, I noticed a big jar of Bag Balm on the shelf. Now, if you don't know about Bag Balm, you're missing out. It was originally invented as a soothing disinfectant for farmers to treat their cows' udders—hence the name. It's a thick salve like petroleum jelly, and it smells vaguely medicinal. It's not exactly a glamorous product, but when I saw it, I laughed out loud.

I remembered a Christmas season in my early twenties. It was a time of spiritual re-birth for me, and my friend Barbara was a wonderful midwife. We spent long evenings by the fire, drinking wine and philosophizing. We also slathered Bag Balm on one another's feet. It was a form of mutual prayer, of play and comfort. My toes still curl in pleasure when I think of that yuletide memory.

One of the joys of my friendship with Barbara is that we're not prone to obligatory gestures or ritualistic gift exchanges. When I saw that Bag Balm, I knew I had to send it to her. Wrapped elegantly, it cost more to mail it than to buy it—but the delight of sharing that memory and anticipating the way Barbara would smile at that unlikely gift, is what Christmas is about for me.

It's a thief in the night. It's accidental joy. And—thank goodness—it will be over soon enough.

Questions for Reflection:

1. What are the ways that joy claims you in the midst of a hectic season? Record in your journal the unexpected pleasures that come your way as you make your way through the holidays.

2. As you shop for gifts, watch for quirky unexpected tokens that have meaning just for the ones on your list. Don't look at price tags. Instead, think of memories you cherish. A card with just the right phrase or

image that evokes a special memory can be much more thoughtful than an expensive pre-wrapped gift from the mall.

3. Consider ways you might resist the tedium of traditional expectations. Spend a day during the Christmas holidays in a stationary shop, browsing for birthday cards for your loved ones throughout the coming year. Arrange them in a calendar or file system to remember each occasion. It will be a holiday gift you give to yourself, and a wonderful way of remembering the year-round blessings of your friends.

## Chapter 49: Ficus Tree

She's not very happy about being here. In fact, she's downright angry. She's mad about paying All That Money, about losing control. About things that I can't even name.

I'm driving her back to the old neighborhood today so her longstanding hairdresser can get her ready for Christmas. She's gone to Lewis for ten years, and she wouldn't think of going to anyone else. By the time we snake our way through Atlanta traffic and miss a few turns, we are an hour late for the appointment.

I leave her in the car and run to Lewis's door. "I have Martha Ellen here. I know we're late. She's real sick, and we got lost on the way from the nursing home." I whisper it quickly to assuage any qualms he might have about accommodating a laggard. He welcomes her warmly, seats her in his chair, and begins to work his fingers through the chemotherapy-ravaged fragments of her hair. He passes me a *Brides Magazine* with a sticky-note attached. "Is she aware of her condition?" he's written. "She's never spoken of it." Yes, she's aware. And no, she's not likely to speak of it. I am touched by the gentleness of his manner.

I thank him profusely as we leave—she looks ever so much better. Lying around hospitals throwing up and shedding hair will dehumanize a person considerably. When we settle into a quiet café, I am gratified to see her wolf down a bowl of vegetable soup. The lack of appetite has been worrisome to her. She doesn't want to see herself failing.

I've brought her ficus tree and a string of tiny clear lights. We settle it into a corner of her room. "It's pretty—real pretty," she exclaims softly as the lights begin to twinkle. Her childlike self is peeking through the clouds of despair that have besieged her lately.

She's always been something of a child. Her imagination eased my journey through some difficult formative years. She bought me stuffed animals of every description and smocked velvet dresses at Christmas time. I always gave her chocolate covered cherries in return. Today, I've brought her a big teddy bear and a box of Ensure.

"These Hospice people are too efficient," she announces. I smile to myself. My brothers and I have avoided the "H" word, referring to them instead as the Nursing Service. "They brought in oxygen tanks and a wheelchair and a walker. They said they'd give me morphine for pain, and for me not to worry about a thing. They got in my face and smiled real big. They even sent the chaplain to see me. I don't *want* them in my face. I don't want to talk about anything. . unpleasant."

I sigh with an odd sense of relief. "You don't have to have anything in your face right now. You're the boss. Let's get rid of the things you don't need."

"You know," she continues, falling back on her pillows, "what I really want is to run away from all this. I want to go back to my condominium. I want to get my car serviced. I want to buy groceries and shop at the mall."

"I know. That's what I want for you, too."

She visibly relaxes. I begin to bargain. "If you stay here awhile, we can care for you better. Just spend time with you. That's all we want."

"It's what I want, too," she says softly. "I need you to be here." Her eyes are clear. It's the most direct statement I can ever remember her making.

A spiritual friend asked recently, "Where are the places you feel God inviting you right now?" I was at a loss in that moment. I didn't imagine God inviting me into a nursing home to offer solace to my dying aunt. But this moment of real-ness is holy ground.

I'm thinking about life transitions—of birth and of death. We gather around expectant couples and shower new mothers with gifts and flowers. When a baby is born, we share stories and do laundry. We tiptoe solicitously about the house, tidying up and preparing nutritious snacks while the new mother naps. We ease her transition from one life into another.

When death approaches, we too often retreat. We limit conversation to vapid reassurances, or formulaic exhortations of the five stages of grief. We speak of the need of the dying to "come to terms with" their impending departure, arrogantly assuming that we know what that means. Or we overwhelm them like over-zealous hospice workers. Bringing wheelchairs and walkers and oxygen tanks and morphine to the bedside of a newly-pronounced terminal patient is a little like bringing bicycles and computers to a baby shower. Although such things will eventually be needed, we don't burden new mothers with the accoutrements of challenges to come.

To stay in the present moment while anticipating need is the task we face as we tend one another. It's the holy ground where God invites us into a deepening consciousness of his care.

Questions for Reflection:

1. Good works are found in those places where our spiritual gifts meet the world's needs. In light of that, where do you feel God inviting you right now? For now, try to let go of notions of goodness or obligation; instead, think of things you can do with a spirit of generosity and freedom.

2. We tend to write off people when we learn they are approaching death, but the process of dying is a major developmental transition. As you think of loved ones who are terminally ill, think of supporting them the same way that you would treat a friend who is preparing to make a major move. If the patient is conscious and accessible, give the gift of your time. Play cards, go for a short drive, see a movie, or just sit and share the silence. With an elderly relative, you might spend time looking at old photographs, sharing family stories, or even recording memoirs. If you live some distance away, frequent notes and cards can be comfort. In all these ways, you give your loved one the opportunity to bless your life through the process of their departure.

## Chapter 50: Christmas Week

It's my favorite week of the year. The holiday cacophony has quieted down. The feasts have been prepared and enjoyed. The gifts have been exchanged. And no one has to hear "It's a Holly Jolly Christmas" or "Rockin' around the Christmas Tree" for another eleven months. Life is good.

The holiday's excesses are part of what make the week between Christmas and New Year's Day so delicious. I never see clients in my office this week. Most people don't want to show up for appointments anyway. I know I'll hit the ground running in January, and it's worth putting life on hold.

The season begins on Christmas Eve. After the shopping and the cooking and the wrapping are done, I tell myself I'm too tired to make it to Midnight Mass, but I always find myself sitting in the pew just the same. The little chapel is transformed by candle-light and the fragrance of greenery. Christmas carols are sung—the contemplative, soulful hymns that nourish our souls throughout the year. "Silent Night." "Oh Come All Ye Faithful." "It Came Upon a Midnight Clear." One thing I love about my religious tradition is the subtle musical shift that happens on Christmas Eve. As the minor keys of Advent give way to the major swell of Christmastide, I feel my heart opening, daring to hope again. Maybe it's sheer fatigue. Maybe it's the relief of having all the shopping done, or maybe it's an overdose of pecan pie and eggnog—but I don't really think so. I think the members of my small community peer into one another's faces and see a glimpse of God.

It's the aftermath that I savor the most—this holy week of timelessness before the old year gives way to the new. My family gathers in the evenings around the fire. We play board games. This year, two generations vied against one another in a fierce Trivial Pursuit™ tournament that went on for several nights. During these long evenings, I witness the miracle that my grown children have evolved from self-absorbed teenagers into young adults with their own life pathways and unique relationships with each other. Long years ago when they were young, I naively said to someone, "Most of all, we need to *enjoy* them." In those tender years, I didn't realize how daunting the prospect of enjoying one's children could be—or what a miracle it would be when, years hence, I would gaze into their faces over a board game and smile at who we have become together. Some Christmases haven't been this easy, of course—and I am wallowing in the delight of this one.

Other pleasures are more ordinary. I wake up slowly in the mornings, savoring the winter sunlight streaming through the French doors of my bedroom. I amble to the kitchen for a cup of coffee and then settle back into bed, nestled between the cat purring contentedly to my left, and the tousle-haired husband snoring gently to my right. The bed seems pleasantly overcrowded, but somehow I balance my journal and my prayer-book and my novel on the mounds of pillows that surround me. I turn from one to the other, recording my dreams and praying the Psalms and immersing myself in stories. I'll go for a walk later this morning, before lunch. I'll stop on my way home to admire the pansies I planted beneath the apple tree in my yard. Their upturned faces always remind me of small children.

I didn't always know to enjoy these pleasures. In my younger years I spent this week dismantling Christmas trees, frantically getting organized and making plans for the New Year. This year I laugh about resolutions. I might dye my hair red this year, I jokingly say to friends. I'll surely develop a more legible handwriting. I'll never forget anyone's birthday, I won't lose my temper, and I'll entertain with more panache. Resolutions are usually stories we tell ourselves—midwinter diversions, nothing more.

Sometimes we are fine, just the way we are. No grand changes are needed.

Questions for Reflection:

1. In what ways do you enjoy your life just the way it is? What are the pleasures that sustain you?

2. This week, take some time for some sensual pleasures. Find an afternoon to take a nap. Savor the taste of your favorite dessert. Notice the subtleties of the season as you step outside to get the newspaper—moist air against your skin, or the rush of the wind on a winter's day. Take a warm bath and slather yourself with your favorite body lotion. Stretch out on freshly washed sheets.

# Chapter 51: Birth Announcement

When I checked my email at dawn today, the computer practically sang out the news. My friend Lynn has become a grandmother. She's ecstatic, of course. I anticipate sharing pictures and stories of each milestone—not only of this baby of hers, but of Lynn herself as she grows into grandmother-hood.

I remember once reading, "Whenever a child is born, so is a mother." It's true. When we bring babies into the world, we birth ourselves as mothers. What we don't know until later is that with the birth of each child, a grandmother, too, is born.

Young motherhood brings a world of wonder. I vividly remember a sense of Divine presence as I noticed the sunlight slanting through the nursery blinds, making halos of my little one's golden curls as she took her afternoon nap. I smelled it in her sweet baby-scent as I rocked her at night before bedtime. "Moments Draped in Bliss," Lisa Groen Braner calls them in *The Mother's Book of Well-Being*.

But motherhood also brings a world of other things—exhaustion, worry, anxiety, and self-doubt. There is no way to do motherhood right. We spend half a lifetime learning that truth through the futile effort of trying to accomplish the impossible. About the time our children are teenagers, we fall back, panting with defeat and confusion. Where did we go wrong? Our intentions were so good. How could we have raised such ill-tempered or defiant or even hostile kids? We scrutinize our choices.

Should we have been more heavy-handed? More understanding? More vigilant in perceiving the signs that our sweet babies were turning into demons before our very eyes?

As we forgive ourselves for having been human, we relax enough to notice that our young adult children have been following a path uniquely their own. If we have given them a modicum of permission to separate from us and be themselves, we find they have learned to listen to the voice of their own truth. An awakening happens when a mother appreciates her children as autonomous individuals with gifts and insights, blind spots and quirks, and passions that are fully their own.

If we are lucky, grandmother-hood comes with this knowledge in tow. Our grown children—hopefully self-sufficient by now—present us with grandchildren. We gaze into the face of a new tiny miracle, and then we look into the eyes of a young parent with a lifetime of hard work and learning ahead.

Grand-mothering brings a new kind of wonder. Having raised children, we know we can't do it right. We don't even have to try. Since there is no injunction to be perfect, we can slow down and do what we do best. If we are gardeners, we teach our grandkids to love the earth. If we are cooks, we bake cookies with them. If we love music, we share singing and dancing. And if we're none of the above, we simply enjoy them.

Enjoying children creates grandmotherly magic. To be successful, children need structure and discipline and affection and routine. They need good nutrition and fresh air and sunshine. They need solid role models and intellectual stimulation. But, even in the absence of some of these essentials, what matters in whether a child succeeds or fails is the presence of at least one person who loves unconditionally—who sees potential and admires accomplishments. Teachers and therapists and siblings can provide this ingredient, but grandmothers are often excellent candidates for the job.

Unconditional love, too, must extend to our own children. Young parents can easily feel abandoned or sabotaged when well-meaning grandparents are critical of their efforts. Although we won't always agree with our adult children, we affirm them and support their growing skills when we respect their parenting styles. In order to do this with authenticity, we have to let go of old roles and rules and stay open to new information. This letting-go and staying-open takes great courage for most of us. Grand-mothering is not for the faint-hearted, and it's definitely not for the young.

I hear Lynn's news with a sense of excitement. She will make a magnificent grandmother. Then I look again at my own grandchildren. They are fully themselves, unspoiled by the world; with them I am recalled to a place where everyday things are enchanting—where possibilities are endless, and stories live and breathe, just waiting to be told.

Questions for Reflection:
1. Write a note to your grandchildren, present or future, and place it in the care of someone who can deliver it to them in the future. Tell them

something about your hopes and dreams for them. Include a few stories about what you treasure the most about them now.

2. This week, try to tune in to each grandchild individually. A quick phone call to hear about their day, or a trip to a museum, or an hour at the park can create warm memories.

3. Make sure you encourage your own children, too. Notice some ways they excel as parents, and tell them about the things you admire. Let go of any temptation to criticize or correct them. Your job now is to support them in every way you can.

## Chapter 52: Wise Blood

The "M" word. Menopause. Sometimes I get tired of hearing it. Go to any doctor with any complaint from headaches to constipation, and you'll hear the word three or four times in the first ten minutes. "It's common in menopause. . ." your (usually male) gynecologist will begin. "Menopausal women tend to . ." "This is just a normal part of menopause." I swear sometimes I could go into a doctor's office and set my hair on fire. He'd peer over the rims of his reading glasses, nod gravely, and sigh with a blend of resignation and reassurance: "Yes. This, too, happens in menopause."

It's not really the word I object to. It's a valid term denoting a major transition. But I do have a problem when the "M" word is used to trivialize inner experience. I flinch when menopause is treated like a disease that plagues the poor woman audacious enough to have lived beyond her prime. And consider the word "prime" here, too. Webster's New World Dictionary defines it as "1. the first or earliest part. 2. the most vigorous period. 3. the best part." The prime of life is often seen as the years when we produce children or contribute the most to the Gross National Product—when we are fruitful in a worldly way.

The ancients had a different understanding. They believed that, during the Change, the blood that had nurtured babies during the childbearing years stayed in the womb to nourish a woman's growing wisdom—hence the term "wise blood." Old women were venerated in indigenous cultures. Their prayers were vital to the health of the tribe. Their counsel was crucial in discerning right action, and their gifts as midwives and healers empowered young women to move into the mysteries of adult femininity.

A popular novel called *The Red Tent* created quite a stir several years back. It's story of biblical times, seen through the eyes of women characters—a perspective too often neglected. The notion that captured the imagination of readers was the red tent itself—a place where women secluded themselves, protected from the cares of the mundane world, during the times of feminine mystery. During menstruation, pregnancy, childbirth, and menopause, women cared for one another. They braided one another's hair and rubbed each other's feet with oil. Old women shared secrets and stories known only within the privacy of that sacred space. Younger ones were comforted.

Red Tent space is sorely lacking today. The last generation's much-touted sexual revolution has cast a pretty dark shadow. The mysteries of femininity and the pleasures of deep intimacy have been splattered into sensationalized images that arouse titillation mixed with aversion, the antithesis of feminine mystery. Most women I know are uncomfortable with the trend, but we want to be "cool," so we allow ourselves and our children to be violated by what amounts to a pornographic assault—the objectification of our innermost selves.

I don't want to sound like a prude; I'm glad that we can talk openly about sexuality. But when I think of kids being regularly exposed to graphic television renditions of incest and rape, I wonder. Where's the real liberation? We're slaves to the very brutality against women that our foremothers protested when Margaret Sanger braved prison to fight for birth control, when Susan B. Anthony endured bodily threats to campaign for women's suffrage.

I'm not naïve enough to want to turn back the clock. But Wise Blood calls us to remember our heritage as midwives and birth-givers. We give birth to children in our younger years. As we enter into the Change, we give birth to visions and dreams for our tribe. We give birth to our own gifts as they manifest in the world, and we midwife the gifts and the dreams of others.

Questions for Reflection:

1. Where is the "red tent" space in your life? In the sauna? In a support group? In a spiritual community? Cultivate your awareness of the gift of that sacred space, and share it as a gift to others.

2. This week, notice the opportunities that arise for you to be a mentor or a role model for younger women. Acknowledge a special event—the anniversary of a baptism, perhaps, or the knowledge that a young friend has entered into womanhood through the menarche—the beginning of menstruation. Write a note, give a gift, or light a candle in honor of that young woman and her gifts.

# Resources

Andrews, Ted (1993), Animal Speak. St. Paul: Llewellyn.

Aizenstat, Stephen Dream-Tending (audiocassette). Boulder: Sounds True.

Arrien. Angeles (1993), The Four-Fold Way. San Francisco: HarperSanfrancisco

Bolen, Jean Shinoda (2001), Goddesses in Older Women. New York: HarperCollins

Boynton, Kim (2003), Zen for Christians. San Francisco: Jossey-Bass.

Braner, Lisa Groen (2003), The Mother's Book of Well Being. York Beach: Conari.

Carter, Cindy (2001), Quetzlcoatl and Tescodlypoca, unpublished manuscript.

Carter, Cindy, (2003), The Seven Individual Rights of Individuality. Santa Barbara, CA: Self- published manuscript.

Connelly, Dianne (1986), All Sickness is Homesickness. Columbia, MD: Center for Traditional Acupucture.

Daimant, A. (1997), The Red Tent. New York: Picador.

Fensterheim, H. (1975), <u>Don't Say Yes When You Want to Say No</u>. New York: Random House.

Friday, N. (1977), <u>My Mother, Myself</u>. New York: Dell.

Hamilton, E. (1942), <u>Mythology</u>. New York: Mentor.

Huddleston, P. (2002), <u>Prepare for Surgery, Heal Faster</u>. Angel River Press.

Hurst, C. (1999), <u>For Mothers of Difficult Daughters</u>. New York: Random House.

Lawrence, B. (reprint ed. 1999), <u>The Practice of the Presence of God</u>. Revell.

Linn, Dennis, et.al. (1999), <u>Healing the Purpose of Your Life</u>. New York: Paulist Press.

Louden, Jennifer (1992), <u>The Woman's Comfort Book</u>. San Francisco: Harper San Francisco.

Merton, T. (1977), <u>New Seeds of Contemplation</u>. New Directions.

Myss, C. (2001), <u>Sacred Contracts</u>. New York: Harmony.

Nemeth, A. (1999), <u>The Energy of Money</u>. New York: Ballantine.

Northrup, C. (2001), <u>The Wisdom of Menopause</u>. New York: Bantam.

Perera, S. (1981), Descent to the Goddess. Toronto: Inner City.

Rilke, R.M. (reissued 2004), Letters to a Young Poet. New York: W.W. Norton.

Rohr, R .(2003), Everything Belongs. New York: Crossroad.

Snowdon, David (2002), Aging with Grace. New York: Bantam.

Smith, M. (1975), When I Say No I Feel Guilty. New York: Bantam.

The Book of Common Prayer. New York: Oxford Press.

von Franz, M.-L. (1974), Shadow and Evil in Fairly Tales. Dallas: Spring.

Woolf, V. (1929), A Room of One's Own. New York: Harcourt Brace Javonovich.

# About the Author

Daphne Stevens, Ph.D., LCSW is a psychotherapist who holds graduate degrees from University of Georgia and Pacifica Graduate Institute. Her dissertation, *Psyche's Plea: Premenstrual Syndrome and the Cultural Betrayal of the Feminine*, was a cross-cultural exploration of women's health and spirituality, and she has been published in print and on-line magazines.

Daphne's work weaves together themes of spirituality, relationships, creativity, and finding the hidden gifts within the experience of grief. Her soul is nourished as a wife and friend, encouraged as a mother and grandmother, and deepened through meditation and spiritual direction. She lives in Georgia with her husband.

For more information, or to contact Daphne, please visit her web site at www.daphnestevens.com.

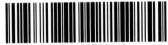

Made in the USA
Columbia, SC
13 February 2018